Humanistic Approaches to Health Care:
Focus on Social Work

Edited by
Norma Berkowitz MSSW

VENTURE PRESS

© British Association of Social Workers, 1996

All rights reserved. No part of this publication may be reproduced, stored in a retrieval system, or transmitted, in any form or by any means, electronic, mechanical, photocopying, recording or otherwise, without the prior permission of Venture Press

Published by
VENTURE PRESS
16 Kent Street
Birmingham
B5 6RD

British Library Cataloguing-in-Publication Data
A catalogue record for this book is available from the British Library

ISBN 1 873878 84 2   (paperback)

Cover design by:
Western Arts
194 Goswell Road
London
EC1V 7DT

Printed and bound in Great Britain by
Biddles Ltd, Guildford and King's Lynn

Contents

	Page
Social Work in a Changing World Series	
Introduction to the series	v
Editor's Introduction	vii
Professor Shulamit Ramon	
Acknowledgements	xiii
The Authors	xv
Rationale for the Structure of this Book	xvii
Chapter 1: Social Work Practice in the Health Care Arena *Norma Berkowitz and Lowell Jenkins*	1
Introduction to the Bio-psychosocial Framework Exemplars	**13**
Chapter 2: Alcohol Abuse: A Bio-psychosocial Perspective *Beverly Flanigan*	15
Chapter 3: Social Work Practice in Hospital Settings: A Bio-psychosocial Perspective *Norma Berkowitz*	33
Chapter 4: Oncology Social Work and Palliative Care in the United States *Matthew J. Loscalzo and James R. Zabora*	49
Introduction to the Public Health Framework Exemplars	**71**
Chapter 5: Primary Health Care: It's Relation to Generalist Practice and to Public Health *Matthew Henk and Louise Doss Martin*	77
Chapter 6: Social Work and Family Planning in Russia: A Public Health Perspective *Natalia Grigorieva*	97
Chapter 7: Public Health and Preventive Strategies: Social Work Practice, HIV Disease and AIDS *Gary A. Lloyd*	113

**Introduction to Strategies for Improving Access,
Utilisation and Quality of Service: Two Examplars**   **129**

Chapter 8: Teams as Means of Interdisciplinary Collaboration:
Developing Community Mental Health in Slovenia   133
Vito Flaker

Chapter 9: Social Work Practice with Refugee Populations in
Hungary: Process and Issues   147
Katalin Talyigas

**Introduction to the Empowerment
Framework Exemplars**   **161**

Chapter 10: Social Work Practice Among Individuals with
Disabling Conditions: An Evolutionary Perspective   165
Mariellen Laucht Kuehn and John W. McClain

Chapter 11: The Empowerment Framework:
Bridging the Gap Between Individuals and
Social Structures in Health Care   181
Audrey Mullender

Chapter 12: Preparing Social Workers for Practice in Health Care   201
Norma Berkowitz and Lowell Jenkins

Appendix A
Disciplinary Contributions to Perspectives on Health Care   217

Social Work in a Changing World Series

Introduction to the series
This series of five books on central aspects of social work and social work education comes as a response to the unprecedented challenges which confront social work as we approach the twenty-first century.

The series was initially commissioned by the Open Society Foundation in Moscow to meet the growing demand for knowledge about social work in the former Soviet Union, where social work is one of the few new professions to emerge in the wake of the defunct Communist era.

Yet it soon became clear to the series editor and the editors of the different volumes that the need for updated, internationally located knowledge and debate about social work is far from being limited to either the former Soviet Union or other east and central European societies. The issues of what is social work, what unifies its ever-increasing diversity, current dominant changes in its knowledge and skills base, the rethinking about clients' and workers' relationships on the one hand and those of social workers, central government and local government on the other hand, and changes in the content and structure of education for social work are British concerns, no less than they are American, Hungarian, Indian, New Zealandian, Portuguese, Russian or South African concerns.

The contributors to the series strongly believe in the potentially positive contribution of social work, as much as they believe in the need to assess its activities critically and to benefit from international perspectives and dialogue while investigating the myriad elements that are social work in a post-modern, post-industrial, post-Communist world.

Up-dated knowledge and information are offered, side by side with a critical analysis of the major changes and challenges to the aspect of social work under consideration.

Written by educators, researchers and workers from ten countries in a jargon-free language, the series presents the latest state of the art. It should be read by anyone interested in social work and concerned about its future.

The volumes published in this series by Venture Press include:

Pathways to Empowerment, edited by Phyllida Parsloe;

Innovations and Continuities in Social Work Education, edited by Shulamit Ramon;

Humanistic Approaches to Health Care: Focus on Social work, edited by Norma Berkowitz;

Social Work with Children and Families: New Directions and Continuing Problems, edited by Judith Harwin;

The Interface between Social Work and Social Policy, edited by Shulamit Ramon.

The series editor is Professor Shulamit Ramon.

Social Work in a Changing World

Editor's Introduction

Since the end of the 1980s we have witnessed considerable political, economic, social and cultural change in east, west, and central Europe.

The scope and depth of change have been particularly dramatic in the former Communist countries, of which Russia is the biggest and the most influential.

These changes have confronted all of us who are interested in the well-being of the citizens of Europe with new, unprecedented challenges.

A number of new groups have become vulnerable in a way they were not before, while the old systems of welfare crumbled and their inability to provide economic, social and psychological safety nets became manifest. This has led to a readiness by policymakers, welfare workers and academics to look for new ways of meeting the emerging needs of such populations. An appetite for learning has been encouraged by eastern Europeans visits to western Europe and the United States, whereby they gained access to some of the experiences and literature available in the West.

At times such visits were all too short; the material looked at not particularly relevant; the cultural differences felt unbridgeable; and issues of power and hegemony too uncomfortable to confront.

Professional social work is one new way of responding to the challenges, obstacles and opportunities presented by these new situations.

There have always been people who helped others informally and formally, such as child care inspectors and social pedagogues who focused on children and recreational activities, but professional social work did not exist in the Soviet Union. In some form social work existed in Czechoslovakia, Romania and Slovenia however.

The uniqueness of social work lies in its attempt to offer a personalised service which holds together the psycho-social levels of our existence. Services are provided by professionally qualified workers who also act as intermediaries between the service user and the State. Usually social workers are not policy makers, though they may - and in my view should - attempt to influence policy decisions. Social workers are accountable to their employers, but their first and foremost loyalty is to defending vulnerable people in our society.

They do so in a variety of ways which are based on knowledge of how people develop, interact, change, learn, become motivated or despair; of how societies influence the lives of individuals; and of how to tread that fragile boundary between influence and coercion and enabling people to determine their choices and to put these into practice.

Social workers are successful at times and unsuccessful at others. Therefore the knowledge of the evaluative evidence on social work is crucial for improving its effectiveness, as well as for ensuring that newcomers to social work will learn from mistakes made in western social work. They will not need to repeat the mistakes but only to make their own, new ones.

An important component of social work is the belief that usually we do not know what is the best choice for another person; that individuals know better than anyone else what is good for them, once they know a lot more about alternative possibilities, the relative advantages and disadvantages of alternative courses of action, and once they have learnt how to make decisions.

This belief contrasts sharply with the view of authoritarian regimes which espouse they have the right to dictate to people what each of them should do individually, and with traditions of top-to-bottom advice giving and handing out of benefits. To acquire the ability to encourage people in a crisis situation to express themselves, to weigh possibilities and to make decisions, and to support them in implementing these decisions, requires not only a non- authoritarian stance but also a genuine belief that all of us have the right and the ability to lead a reasonably satisfactory life, however varied the range of 'satisfactory' must be.

Social work does not exist outside of specific political and cultural contexts. In the west it originated within the context of liberal capitalism. As liberal capitalism is now challenged by the New Right and pro-'free' market orientation western social work finds itself in a serious crisis in terms of adherence to its values, and its conceptual and practice frameworks which come from its previously dominant ideology.

This fact must be baffling for east Europeans impressed by the richness of the fabric of services and professional activities of western social work. In fact they may see the notion of such a 'crisis' as western indulgence.

Often westerners do not share with their eastern European friends their knowledge of this crisis for fear that this may prevent the latter from being interested in social work at all.

Editor's Introduction

The position taken throughout the series SOCIAL WORK IN A CHANGING WORLD is the wish to share our ideas about social work as honestly as possible, warts and all, crisis and disillusionment, in the belief that this is the best way forward for the development of social work, wherever it is taking place.

Therefore, the form which social work should take in any one country has to come out of the context of the specific country; imitation of models of social work used elsewhere is unlikely to work well without such an adaptation.

Yet this series is based on the belief that nevertheless the *core* of social work is international because it is based on *common human experience*, and provides a guide to the content and format of social work in any one country (Midgely and Khinduka, 1992).

That *core* consists first and foremost in social work values (Shardlow, 1989), including:

- the right of individuals to be supported by their communities and societies when facing adversity and becoming vulnerable;
- the right to be treated with respect and be offered dignity;
- the right to self-determination, as long as it does not entail risk to oneself and/or others;
- the right to fail, as well as the right to fulfil one's potential, is an integral component of the right to self- determination.
- the responsibility of individuals for their own actions.

This is followed by the generalised knowledge of:

- how people develop and change;
- the role played by society in such a process;
- how people respond to adversity;
- what helps people in a crisis and what does not;
- what supports people in a way which enables them to take greater control over their own reality and to use their own potential.

The core social work skills which are based on the professional values and knowledge consist in:

- the ability to communicate with people experiencing adversity;
- the ability to form good personalised yet *professional* relationships with clients in which empathy and genuineness are expressed on the one hand, and yet are free from exploitation on the other;
- the ability to connect people to existing networks and create new networks if required;
- the ability to advocate and intermediate;
- knowledge and use of a wide range of formal and informal resources in the community;
- the ability to counsel individuals, families and groups;
- the ability to live with the losses and pain experienced by others without succumbing to the impact of such suffering oneself.
- the ability to reflect on, and evaluate one's own work, and to change it in the light of the lessons thus learnt.

Furthermore, it is productive to learn about how other societies conceptualise and operationalise their social work framework, as such learning generates ideas and helps to prevent the repetition of mistakes.

Reading about different approaches to social work is the least coercive way to influence people interested in learning about social work in post-Communist countries, for it allows them to reflect on what they have read, decide on their own what appeals to them and how to use it.

In social work we believe that *reflection* is indispensable in taking stock of situations and processes, of our own activities and those of others, and as a necessary, but insufficient, condition for the provision of a personalised service (Schon, 1983).

Such a reflection is necessary for negotiating the eternal dilemmas which social workers face constantly. For example, it would be naïve and misleading to suggest that social work is providing support only to people in adversity; it is also one of the more sophisticated tools of social control invented by liberal capitalism.

Social work exercises social control in a variety of ways, exemplified by the coercive form of taking children away from their parents, recommending that people be admitted to psychiatric hospitals, and influencing people's views of themselves and others at the psychological level.

Editor's Introduction

Indeed, the conflict between exercising care and control and the inevitability that care does not come without some type of control is one of the dilemmas which all social workers face in every society.

This dilemma relates to yet another problematic issue; namely with whom does the primary loyalty of the social worker lie: is it with the State? with the specific employer? with the identified client? with the society in which the worker operates? In terms of core social work values, this loyalty has to be first to the client, and then to society, with the loyalty to the employer and the State trailing behind. Such a commitment may be seriously tested at times, and social workers require considerable peer and professional support to stick by the loyalty to the client and to society in general.

A good text on any aspect of social work would need to pay attention to these dilemmas.

The new series is thus dedicated to the coverage of social work values, knowledge and skills, in the context of different needs, wishes, client groups, and social contexts.

It is not accidental that the series forms a part of the activities of the TRANSFORMATION PROJECT OF THE HUMANITIES AND THE SOCIAL SCIENCES of the Soros Cultural Initiatives Foundation in Moscow. It was the initiative of Professor Teodor Shanin - the director of the project until November 1994 - that put social work on the map of the Transformation Project. This alliance with the Russian Ministry of Higher Education has led to the beginning of the dialogue between British, American and Russian social work educators. The initiative has been supported systematically from its inception by the current director of the project, Mr Victor Galizin.

In a number of ways, the move to develop professional social work in post-Communist countries embodies the challenges, opportunities and obstacles with which we are confronted throughout Europe. Particularly in post-Communist societies. Social work challenges traditional beliefs on the relationships between citizens and officialdom; the role of officialdom; the rights and responsibilities of individuals versus, the rights and duties of the State; the relationships between individuals and their communities; the abilities and potential of vulnerable people; the often fragile balance between the rational and the emotional components of our existence; care and control; and the nature of professionalism (Payne, 1991).

Thus it befits the Transformation Project, dedicated to introducing tools to facilitate transformation in the Humanities and the Social Sciences, to include the introduction of social work as a social science discipline as one of its core activities.

Professor Shulamit Ramon
series editor

References

Midgely, J. Khinduka, S. Hokenstad, M. (eds.) (1992) *International Profiles of Social Work*, American Social Workers Association, Washington, D.C.

Payne, M. (1991) *Modern Social Work Theory: A Critical Introduction*, Macmillan, London.

Schon, D. (1983) *The Reflective Practitioner: How professionals think in action*, Basic Books, New York.

Shardlow, S. (1989) (ed.) *The Value of Change in Social Work*, Routledge, London.

Acknowledgements

The satisfaction of having produced a book which may be helpful to others is accompanied by the feeling of gratitude for those who made it possible.

I am indebted to Professor Shulamit Ramon for the opportunity to engage in the task and to the authors who committed their words and wisdom to paper within a constricted timetable and in the midst of already busy professional lives.

Special thanks are extended to Bradford Sheafor who provided consultation and direction in use of the Teaere and Sheafor as yet unpublished data on manpower; to the School of Social Work for the support of Carol Grogan, who provided editing assistance; and Ruth Evans, administrative staff, who kept faxes efficiently traversing the country and the ocean.

Two publishing organisations gave permission for use of previously published material. Sage Publications, London, for use of material which previously appeared on pp. 55 - 66 in the book *Social Work in Primary Care* by Matthew Henk (1989). Massachusetts General Hospital's Institute on the Health Professions gave permission to adapt material from their publication *Development of Health Social Work Curricula: Patterns and Process in Three Programs of Social Work Education*; edited by Barbara Berkman and Thomas Owen Carlton (1985).

Ongoing support from my husband, Leonard Berkowitz, and his patient assistance in enabling me to use computer technology, helped this project become reality.

The authors

Norma Berkowitz: MSSW, Emeritus Faculty, School of Social Work, University of Wisconsin-Madison, USA.

Vito Flaker: Co-ordinator TEMPUS Programme in Training for Psycho-Social Services, Assistant Lecturer, School of Social Work, University of Ljublijana, Ljublijana, Slovenia.

Louise Doss-Martin: M.A.; Senior Social Work Consultant, United States Public Health Service, Bureau of Primary Health Care, Washington, D.C.

Beverly Flanigan: MSSW, Clinical Professor, School of Social Work, University of Wisconsin-Madison, USA.

Natalia Grigorieva: Social Science and Ph. D. Natural Sciences, Moscow State University, Centre for Development and Population Activities, Moscow; Vice-President of International Women's Centre, Moscow.

Matthew Henk: MSW; Public Health Social Work Consultant, United States Public Health Service, Regional Public Health Office, Kansas City, Missouri, USA.

Lowell Jenkins: MSW; Professor of Social Work, Colorado State University, Fort Collins, Colorado, USA.

Mariellen Laucht Kuehn: MSSW, Ph.D., Associate Director of University Affiliated Program, Waisman Centre, University of Wisconsin, Madison, Wisconsin, USA.

Gary Lloyd: Ph.D.; Professor of Social Work, Co-Ordinator of the Institute for Research and Training in HIV\AIDS Counselling, Tulane University School of Social Work, New Orleans, Louisiana, USA.

Matthew Loscalzo: MSW, Director, Oncology Social Work, The John Hopkins Oncology Centre; and Research Associate, The John Hopkins School of Medicine, Baltimore, Maryland, USA.

John W McClain: Ph.D.; Director of the Policy Institute, Meyer Rehabilitation Institute, University Affiliated Program, University of Nebraska Medical School, Omaha, Nebraska, USA.

Audrey Mullender: Professor of Social Work, University of Warwick, Warwick, England.

Katalin Talyigas: Ph.D., Executive Director, Hungarian Jewish Social Support Foundation; Lecturer, Socialpolitical Faculty, the ELTE, University of Budapest, Hungary.

James R. Zabora: MSW; Director of Patient and Family Services, The John Hopkins Oncology Centre; Research Associate, The John Hopkins School of Medicine, Baltimore, Maryland, USA.

Rationale for the Structure of this Book

This book is designed to be an introduction and a tool for use in the education of social pedagogues and social workers in Russia and other parts of the Soviet Union at a time when social work is emerging as a distinct profession. Many people such as volunteers, family members and clergy, provide social help to those in need. However, this book stresses the special contributions that professionally trained social workers make to those individuals, families and groups of people who become ill and/or who suffer from disabling conditions.

The material is presented in a way which promotes a systems and generalist approach to social work practice in health care. The term 'generalist' is used as specifically defined in American literature (and chapter 1 of this book) and readers from other countries are encouraged to relate this concept to the emerging definitions of 'specialist' and 'generalist' and 'social worker' and 'social pedagogue' as used in their own context.

The 'generalist' perspective as used in this book does not preclude the need for 'specialist' social workers in health care settings, but acknowledges that great improvements in the quality of life for those with health-related problems and handicapping conditions can be realised through the efforts of social workers who do not have specialised training in health care and who work in non-medical settings. Social workers in all settings can contribute to the quality of life and maintenance of health of those they serve only if they have an understanding of health care based on a solid philosophical and practice theory.

Those social workers with specialised training in health social work may best be utilised in highly specialised settings, working with complex populations with specialised and complicated medical and social needs. They may also be most effective in programme and policy formulation, administration and research.

The authors acknowledge tensions which exist at the interface between social services and the medical and health care cultures. We live in a time when the science of a profession is lauded more than its humanism. Social workers involved in serving those who are ill or have disabling conditions often work collaboratively with medical personnel whose primary values are reflected in science and technology. The profession of social work itself experiences consistent tension regarding the degree of impact that scientific findings and humanistic values should have on practice.

This book stresses a humanistic approach to practice which is guided by theoretical knowledge gleaned from the scientific method of research. However, the approach is 'client centred', whether the 'client' (the one seeking social work assistance) is an individual, group, organisation, community, or identified 'population at risk'. The book addresses the system of delivering health care as well as the social worker's direct involvement in providing service to those with health-related problems.

Another tension underlying the provision of health-related services is the tension between institutional and community care. Who requires care in medical facilities? To what extent can medical needs be addressed in community social settings and thereby improve the quality of life of many people suffering from chronic or disabling conditions?

The various exemplars address another tension, that of what is 'social' and what is 'medical'. Both the social worker and the medical professionals involved in providing services to those with illnesses and disabilities must constantly manage this tension in order to assure appropriate and adequate delivery of services. Wherever and however services are provided, they ideally include attention to the biological, psychological, and social dimensions of human existence.

The book stresses the process and problem-solving orientation that is characteristic of all social work practice. The exemplars identify contemporary social problems and the roles and interventions which professional social workers utilise in addressing these problems. Each section of the book is preceded by a brief summary of a framework relevant to addressing the problem presented.

Chapter 1 discusses the social context for social work in health care and presents practice perspectives useful for meeting the challenges to practitioners in any arena of practice which addresses health-related problems.

Chapters 2, 3 and 4, are exemplars focusing on the bio-psycho-social framework that is crucial to social work practice in the health care arena. Chapters 5, 6 and 7 provide exemplars focusing on health-related problems in the context of a public health framework.

Chapters 8 and 9 identify strategies which social workers employ to assure access, quality, and/or utilisation of social work services in health-related practice.

Chapters 10 and 11 present two perspectives on empowerment and the strategies social workers have evolved to help those with disabling conditions gain some power and control over their lives.

Rationale for the Structure of this Book

The final chapter briefly summarises the book's content and notes the utilisation of social workers in health care in the United States. The chapter concludes with an exploration of the curriculum content needed to prepare social workers for meeting the needs of those with health-related problems as they encounter them in their practice.

References

Bocharova, Valentina; *Social Work in Russia* Materials for the International Social Work Seminar; (1993). Association of Social Pedagogues and Social Workers of Russia; Moscow.

Schatz, Mona; Jenkins, Lowell; Sheafor, Bradford; 'Milford Redefined: A Model of Initial and Advanced Generalist Practice', *Journal of Social Work Education;* Vol. 26, 3 (Fall) (1990). Wash., D.C. Council on Social Work Education.

Chapter 1
Social Work Practice in the Health Care Arena
Norma Berkowitz and Lowell Jenkins

Introduction

'Illness is the night-side of life... Everyone who is born holds dual citizenship in the kingdom of the well and in the kingdom of the sick.' Although we all prefer to maintain ourselves in the 'kingdom of the well', most of us sooner or later spend some time in the 'kingdom of the sick'. Yet even as we inhabit the kingdom of the well, we are haunted by the fantasies, myths and misconceptions about those who, either for a short time or a long time, sporadically or continuously, cope with living in the 'kingdom of the sick' (Sontag, 1990).

Every society that claims to be civilised and based on humanitarian principles has been concerned with those who enter the 'kingdom of the sick'. Sometimes this concern has been addressed by ecclesiastical bodies who even in medieval times freely admitted the weak, sick, and disabled to monastic hospitals. Sometimes it was the aristocracy, hoping to secure their place in contemporary society as well as in 'the future life', who served the 'kingdom of the sick' through philanthropy and 'good works'. Sometimes, as in modern welfare societies, it is the State itself which assumes the primary task of providing for such citizens.

The social work profession has a long and complicated history of service to both kingdoms. Its history is that of a humane profession, characterised by an emphasis on humanistic values and concerns. However, the social work profession shares with ecclesiastical bodies altruistic values and deep commitment to serve and care for those who are ill and those with handicapping conditions which render them vulnerable to disease. Indeed, the very word 'profession' has its etymological roots in 'the act of openly declaring', and 'professing' oneself to 'uphold the vows of a religious order'.

Today social workers serving those in the kingdom of the sick still function in hospitals, hospices, special schools and institutions affiliated with ecclesiastical bodies.

The social work profession shares with philanthropy a humanitarian perspective, a concern for human welfare, and the promotion of social reforms. The current emphasis on social work involvement in the development of non-governmental organisations, which derive both their funding and their social reform mission from philanthropic individuals and foundations, is a current manifestation of these ties. Such philanthropic activities in the United Kingdom and the United States gave birth to social work education and to the establishment of the social work profession in medical settings devoted to treating those who were ill and rehabilitating those suffering from disabling conditions.

Social work as a profession has a complex relationship with the State in that it benefits from the legitimation bestowed on it by the State. But at the same time it suffers from limitations imposed on it by state Statutes, policies and legislation. Social service systems have been integrated with the government's mission to provide concrete goods and services to vulnerable populations such as those who are poor or ill, have long-term chronic conditions and disabilities and are discriminated against because of race, colour or creed. The professions role then becomes extremely complex and needs constant assessment and monitoring. A strong professional organisation, coalitions with other professions, a commitment to advocacy and social reform, and alliances with consumer groups are strategies often used to protect the modern profession of social work from being co-opted by the State. These strategies also help the profession retain its mission to serve those vulnerable populations and individuals in need of health care and a variety of other social services.

The relationship of the profession to those who inhabit the 'kingdom of the well' is less well established, even though the professions commitment to the well is embedded in its social reform history. These reforms were dedicated to keeping people well and preventing them from becoming ill as a result of poor sanitation and housing, exposure to infectious disease, poverty, lack of immunisation and of access to medical care. In the United States, the experience of Jane Addams, founder in 1893 of the Hull House Settlement for immigrants to Chicago, provided the framework for this orientation to the profession (Addams,1910, 1945).

By 1927 the contributions of social work practice to public health were recognised in the United States when social workers were included in the tuberculosis programme of a large metropolitan county public health department in the USA.

While still adhering to this public health commitment, contemporary social work practice in the United States addresses new concerns with those inhabiting the 'kingdom of the well'. Epidemiological data indicate that life-style choices, environmental hazards and ways of coping with life's emergencies and losses greatly affect one's vulnerability to disease. Social workers today play a major counselling role designed to assist people in developing and maintaining healthy life-styles and positive mental attitudes. They also assume a major educative and activist role designed to modify environments which may increase the potential for acquiring illness and/or disabling conditions. They increasingly provide health education and health promotion information using group interventions and mass media.

Social Work Practice in the Health Care Arena

As a profession, social work performs two major functions in relation to problems related to wellness, illness and disability:

(1) it spans the boundary between disease oriented medical disciplines and humanistically oriented social science disciplines (such as psychology, sociology and anthropology) and between the bureaucracies of health and social welfare services;

(2) it encourages and maintains a focus on the impact of the social environment and adverse social conditions on the prevention, treatment and rehabilitation of those served by the health care system.

The Social Context of Health Care

The delivery of services to promote health care and to mediate health problems takes place in a social context. Too frequently both the general public and the health professions think of health care in the limited sense of curing disease and providing medical care to those in institutions and facilities manned by medical scientists who follow the scientific method in isolating and treating disease entities which have invaded the human body. This may be called the *residual* approach to health care.

The mission of those involved in the provision of 'health care,' however, is much broader and requires a perspective which goes beyond a disease orientation. There are two reasons for this. Topliss, among others, has pointed out that the greatest potential for the diminution of ill-health lies in prevention at a personal level by the adoption of healthier ways of life (Topliss, 1978). Such an approach offers social workers an opportunity to provide an important educational function focused on health promotion and health maintenance, to individuals, families and groups.

Secondly, the very successes of medical science in reducing the toll of diseases, conditions and accidents that used to be lethal for lower-age groups, has left a population of survivors likely to be beset by longer-term, less soluble problems. Topliss maintains, therefore, that health services will need to develop an overwhelming emphasis on care rather than cure (Topliss, 1978).

It is in the light of this latter development that both medical and social work practice must adapt. This population requires long term continuity of care, experiences periodic hospitalisation and episodic acute care incidents, and must be carefully monitored and managed. The needs of this group go far beyond the traditional requirements for medication. They require health care delivery systems that bridge the gap between medical and social services and between the provision of care in hospitals and care in the community. Medical and social work practitioners must have substantive collaboration and effective partnerships based on mutual understanding of and respect for each other's contributions if this population is to be treated effectively, humanely and with dignity. It is this population which society often isolates, neglects and stigmatises. It is this population which many social workers will most frequently serve in their everyday practice and whose medical and social needs require frequent assessment and adjustment.

Definitions of health vary across time and cultures. Anderson (1984) has devised a classification system of health definitions and he points out that health is variously defined: (1) as a product or outcome of some activity; (2) as a capacity to achieve preferred goals or perform certain functions; (3) as a process whereby health is an ever-changing dynamic phenomenon; (4) as something experienced by individuals; (5) as an attribute of an individual (for example, physical fitness), or as a characteristic of the whole person (for example, emotions).

Those trained in scientific medicine may well define health as 'the absence of disease or biological disturbance' (Calnan, 1987). However, lay people generally tend to say they are healthy if they are able to carry out their daily routine, in spite of the medical, social and sometimes technological support they may require to do so.

The most idealistic definition of health, and one which guides some countries and organisations in setting goals relative to health care, is one proposed by the World Health Organization in 1948: 'Health is a state of complete physical, mental and social well-being.'

Whatever definition of health one favours, or however a government or profession operationalises it, it is clear that social factors weigh heavily in the definition, as well as in the perceptions and values underlying the definition.

On a societal level, health-related professions often claim exclusive right to serve, or refuse to serve, categories of people who are ill or have handicapping conditions. Ideologies, cultural beliefs and stereotypes as well as economic realities influence how governments perceive and provide for a nation's state of health and well-being.

On an individual level, it has been suggested that patterns of health and illness behaviour are associated with types of family structure such as the marital relationship, the structure of social networks and parental child-rearing patterns (Pratt, 1976).

Individual membership in a particular sub-group of a society also affects health status. Based on extensive research findings, Falck indicates that gender, age or life stage, family and other social relationships, membership in a racial/ethnic group, social class, occupation, and mental status are important variables which can affect health status (Falck, 1981).

Early social work pioneers in medical social work in the United States identified a number of 'adverse social factors associated with individual problems of ill health': adverse factors affecting subsistence (such as inadequate physical protection); inadequate economic protection; faulty health habits; dissatisfaction with family/group relationships; dissatisfaction connected with restricted outlets (Thornton, 1937).

Two thorough reviews of the social work research literature in the United States in 1978 (Berkman, 1978; Bracht 1978) supported the premise that social, cultural and economic conditions have a significant and measurable effect on both health status and illness prevention and that social work interventions in these areas can be effective.

Social Work Roles and Functions

Disease is something an *organ* has; illness is something a *man* has' (Gelman, 1981). This is an important distinction for those social workers whose practice involves working directly with people who have a health-related problem. It is particularly significant to those working in medical settings staffed primarily by medical doctors.

Societies at various times and in various places have bestowed the responsibility for curing disease on witch doctors, shamans, ecclesiastics, and faith healers. In most industrialised societies in modern times, this responsibility falls to medical doctors and physicians trained in scientific medicine, who utilise the methods of natural science.

Part of the role confusion experienced by social workers in health care may lie in the fact that the entities called 'disease' and 'illness' are conceptually distinct but the relationship between the two is neither simple nor generally understood (Calnan, 1987).

Disease is defined as an abnormal condition of an organism, or specific part of an organism, that impairs normal physiological functioning, especially as a result of infection, inherent weakness, or environmental stress (Webster 1984).

Contemporary definitions of *illness*, however, focus on the of evaluating bodily changes and the decision-making process which results in a person being assigned to, or assigning themselves to the sick role. 'Becoming ill' in this sense is a *process*, one in which the affected person notices symptoms, labels them, decides what to do about them, and then, finally, makes a decision about whether or not they are *ill*.

Part of the role ambiguity experienced by medical doctors in relation to the management of social factors affecting health status may be attributed to the fact that there is considerable difference in the way lay people and medical doctors define 'illness'. Lay people perceive illness as a state of being which interrupts their perceived relationship with their bodies and a state which negatively affects their ability to carry on their daily lives. Medical doctors, on the other hand, tend to perceive people who are ill as those suffering from disease. Medical practitioners, therefore predominantly tend to focus on organs and organicity, while people who are 'ill' tend to focus on how they feel and on the disruption in daily living and functioning caused by feeling un-well (Calnan, 1987).

The social work profession has never claimed that curing disease is a function or goal of social work practice! However, social workers have historically played an important role in helping individuals and families deal with the social and psychological consequences of illness and disability in their daily lives. The term 'disability' is used in this context to refer to the sense of being incapacitated or in a disabled state that restricts or prevents normal achievement.

Social workers dealing with health-related issues in their practice are bound by the same purposes and functions that are the foundation of all social work. The purpose of social work and the unique mission of the profession was stated by Minahan and Pincus when they noted that social workers seek to promote or restore a mutually beneficial interaction between individuals and society in order to improve the quality of life for everyone (Minahan and Pincus, 1977).

The specific purpose of social work in (relation to) health is to provide professional services to people whose ability to function socially in community with others is disrupted, or may be disrupted, by illness, disability or injury (Berkman, 1985).

> 'To achieve this purpose, the profession is guided in its work by knowledge of individuals, by knowledge of developmental psychology and human development theories and life-cycle knowledge that covers the individual life span from birth through death' (Rosenberg, 1983).

These statements of purpose emphasise the profession's unique focus on person/environment transactions that are so important to the well-being and quality of life of those who are ill or who suffer from chronic and disabling conditions.

In light of these statements, it is clear that social workers dealing with health-related problems perform tasks for, and provide services to, a wide array of people at various stages of development: children, adolescents, young and mature adults and elderly people. They provide services to individuals with a wide variety of medical conditions, both acute and chronic, with short term and long term consequences. They deal with people in crisis because of traumatic incidents as well as providing solace to those facing death.

Social Work Practice in the Health Care Arena

Social workers deal with health-related problems in the context of practice in nearly every setting: small isolated villages in rural areas; in congested areas of large cities; in shelters, prisons, day care centres, schools and community centres. They also encounter and serve those who are ill and disabled in settings which are primarily medical in nature: hospitals, institutions serving those with severe disabilities, public health clinics and polyclinics and medical practices.

They deal with people whose problems stem primarily from emotional problems and those who have emotional difficulties because of their medical condition.

They serve people who are 'well' by participating in health promotion and education activities in the community. They serve those whose chronic illness makes them dependent on the care of others and who require long-term assistance either at home or in protected settings such as nursing homes, group homes and hospices.

They provide services to those experiencing social-psychological-emotional disequilibrium and interrelationship difficulties arising from health problems. They serve those who have social diseases resulting from lifestyle and environmental factors; diseases such as cirrhosis, emphysema, substance abuse, coronary disorders, sexually transmitted diseases and cancers caused by toxic air, water and food. They encounter those whose health status is affected by social disorders such as war, criminal and domestic violence, and turmoil following natural disasters. They help the 'worried well' and the 'stabilised sick' deal with stress, anxiety and fear that would make them more vulnerable to illness and disease.

The interventions social workers utilise to address health-related concerns may be directed toward an INDIVIDUAL who is experiencing a health-related problem; a GROUP of individuals trying to cope with a specific illness, such as cancer; FAMILIES forced to restructure their roles as the result of a family member's illness; an ORGANISATION striving to serve the needs of a particular population with special health problems; or a COMMUNITY faced with physical, social or environmental problems posing a danger to its residents.

In light of this broad spectrum of populations, problems, and contexts, social work educators have tried to identify the functions and roles assumed by social workers as they address health-related practice issues.

Pincus and Minahan have used a social systems framework for social work practice based on general systems theory (Bertalanffy, 1950). Through use of this analytical model, which can be applied to any instance of the process of social organisation from families to nations, they have identified seven functions which would be applicable to social workers involved in humanistic approaches to health care (Pincus and Minahan, 1973). They are: (1) to help people enhance and more effectively utilise their own problem-solving and coping capacities; (2) to establish initial linkages between people and resource system; (3) to facilitate interaction and modify and build new relationships between people and societal resource systems; (4) to facilitate interaction and modify and build relationships between people within resource systems; (5) to contribute to the development and modification of social policy; (6) to dispense material resources; (7) and as Ramon also has pointed out in the preface to this volume, to act as an agent of social control.

Germain views the major social work function in face-to-face practice in health care as helping those who are ill, and their families, deal with social and emotional needs and problems that may accompany or predate illness and disability (Germaine, 1984). For Germain, improving person-environment relationships by easing associated stress and enhancing internal and external copying resources is central to social work practice in health care. In light of this dual focus, Germaine divides social work roles designed to help clients to cope with the stress of illness, injury or disability into those focused on the CLIENT (mobiliser, teacher, coach, enabler and facilitator) and those focused on the ENVIRONMENT (mobiliser, collaborator, mediator, organiser, facilitator, innovator, advocate). In the mobiliser role the social work task is to provide incentives and rewards for coping. In the teacher, coach, collaborator, mediator roles the task is to provide instruction in coping skills, individually or in groups. As an enabler and organiser, the social work tasks are to provide emotional support, to influence organisations/agencies to respond to emotional needs, and to organise and work with natural support systems. As facilitator, innovator and advocate the social work tasks are to provide information, time and space for effective coping; to provide opportunities for choice, decision making and action; to create new programmes and services to meet new needs; and to influence organisational and other environments to change when needed.

Another way of viewing practice is the 'generalist perspective'. It, too, focuses on the transactions between person and environment and the interface between systems. It provides equal emphasis on the goals of social justice, humanising social systems, and improving the well-being of people. The basic elements in generalist practice include: (1) utilisation of multi-level problem solving methodology; (2) a multiple theoretical orientation which includes an ecological systems model that recognises the interrelatedness of human problems, life situations and social conditions; (3) a knowledge, value and skill base which is transferable between and among diverse contexts, locations and problems; (4) an open assessment not constricted by any particular theoretical or intervention approach; and (5) selection of strategies or roles for intervention which are made on the basis of the problem, goals, and situation demanding attention and the size of the systems involved (Schatz, Jenkins and Sheafor, 1990).

There are also specific characteristic of generalist practice:

(1) Open methodology. The concept implies that social workers must become proficient in various methods of social work activities. They must be able to work with individuals, families, groups, organisations and communities and know how social policy is developed and initiated.

(2) The ideological bases that inform this perspective are democracy, humanism and empowerment.

(3) The perspective demands a multi-level systems assessment and frequently requires multi-level systems interventions. It requires sequential or simultaneous interventions, often using more than one mode of practice, with various-sized systems.

(4) The generalist must have the ability to function in varied practice roles, including that of broker, advocate, mediator, educator, social activist, and clinician.

(5) The perspective requires a client-centred approach in which the client's goals are paramount.

(6) The social work process is focused on mutually-agreed-upon goals and steps toward problem solving, with the social worker responsible for managing the use of time so that the potential inherent in each phase of the process, and in the process as a whole, may be fully realised for the client (Carlton, 1984).

(7) The generalist social worker employs a research base to inform and guide practice.

(8) The generalist must have the competence to function within the environment of a social agency.

(9) The generalist must be a 'reflective practitioner', be able and willing to examine and to evaluate his or her own practice either independently or within a supervisory or consultative relationship. This may require competency in designing survey instruments, engaging in content analysis of recordings and records, and using other existing tools for self-assessment.

The systems and ecological approaches to practice, combined with the generalist perspective, provide a potent framework for practice within medical and health-related settings and with those who are ill or disabled. Most importantly, the generalist perspective complements the holistic and existential dimensions which are so critical to health-related practice.

This holistic approach, based on common, basic human needs implies: (1) the need to love and be loved; (2) the need to relate to others; (3) the need to have material needs met, and (4) the need to develop to maturity and to achieve maximum personal growth.

The foundation for this approach to practice, however, is embedded in the values and philosophy, the knowledge base, the identified competencies, the professional mission, the public legitimation of the profession (from government, legally incorporated private agencies, clients and consumers) and the ethical principles for practice which the profession has adopted. (Sheafor, Horejsi and Horejsi, 1988).

The Social Work Process
The idea of process refers to 'life flow'. All life is in process, whether it is a cell, an organ, a human being, a family, a group, an organisation, a community, a society or a country. All social work practice involves process since it involves intervening in this 'life flow'. When social workers intervene in this 'life flow', they become engaged in a change process designed to address some presenting problem.

A recent study in the United States compared components of this problem-solving, or change, process as identified in social work literature. It is noted that although the labels vary, the following phases in this process are common to all practice approaches that the social worker should master: (1) intake and engagement; (2) data collection and assessment; (3) planning and contracting; (4) intervention and monitoring; and (5) evaluation and termination, (Sheafor, Horejsi and Horejsi, 1988).

This process is recognised as a dynamic one in which there may be both growth and regression before a final synthesis or internalised growth is achieved.

Most often the social worker involved in health care will enter the life space of an individual or family when the life flow has been disrupted because of injury- or illness- related incidents which disrupt the usual activities of daily living and social and role relationships. In light of this, new problems in living arise. These must be resolved by engaging in some type of problem-solving process either alone or with family members and friends or with health professionals.

When professional social workers become engaged in this problem-solving process with an individual or family, organisation or community, there is the expectation that, by working together there can be movement toward planned change, that mutually identified problems can move toward resolution and that movement toward mutually agreed upon goals may be realised.

At the heart of this planned change process is the relationship between social worker and client. And at the heart of this relationship are the democratic and humanist values of the social worker which facilitate development of a trusting relationship based on mutuality and respect.

Development of a mutually defined 'programme for work', often referred to as a 'contract' or an 'intervention plan', between worker and client, maximises the potential for successful outcomes to the problem-solving process. Basic to problem-solving ideology are the philosophical views of existentialism. It is assumed that all of human life is engaged in a natural struggle toward the goal of better adaptation. The approach suggests that people, individually and collectively, can alter their own behaviour if they possess a clear idea of what to do and if their wishes regarding problem definition are respected (Abrams, 1983). The problem-solving process views people as capable of acting in a responsible, independent manner in their own behalf, including making decisions about their health maintenance and, in concert with health professionals, management of their health-related problems.

References

Abrams, Sandra (1983) in Carol Meyer (ed.) *Clinical Social Work in the Eco-Systems Perspective*; NY; Columbia University Press.

Addams, Jane (1910, 1945). *Twenty Years at Hull House*. NY Macmillan.

Anderson, R. (1984). Health Promotion: An Overview; European Monograph's in *Health Education Research* 6: 4-119.

Berkman, Barbara (1978). *Social Work and Health Care: A Review of the Literature*; Chicago; Society for Hospital Social Work.

Berkman, Barbara and Owen, Carleton (eds) (1985). "Development of a Health - Social Work Curricula: Patterns and Process" in *Three Programs of Social Work Education* ; Boston: Institute of Health Professions, Mass. General Hospital.

Bertalanffy, Ludwig Von (1950). 'An Outline of General Systems Theory'; *British Journal for the Philosophy of Science*; Vol.1, 1950.

Bracht, Neil F. (1978) *Social Work in Health Care: A Guide to Professional Practice*; NY; Haworth Press.

Calnan, Michael (1987). *Health and Illness: The Lay Perspective*; London,Tavistock Pub. Ltd.

Carlton, Thomas Owen (1984). *Clinical Social Work in Health Settings;* NY; Springer.

Falck, Hans S. (1981) *The Social Status Exam in Health Care*; Richmond; School of Social Work, Virginia Commonwealth University.

Gelman, C.; (1981) 'Disease Versus Illness in General Practice'; *Journal of Royal College of General Practice* 31:548-52.

Germaine, Carel Bailey (1984) *Social Work Practice in Health Care: An Ecological Perspective*; NY; Free Press.

Minahan, Anne and Pincus, Allen (1973) "Conceptual Frameworks for Social Work Practice"; *Social Work Journal* Volume 22 issue 5 September 1977.

Pratt, L. (1976) *The Energized Family: Family Structure and Effective Health Behavior*; Houghton Mifflin, Boston.

Rosenberg, Gary (1983) *Advancing Social Work Practice in the Health Care Field*; (eds) Rosenberg, Gary and Rehr, Helen; NY; Haworth Press.

Schatz, Mona; Jenkins, Lowell; Sheafor, Bradford *'Milford Redefined: A Model of Initial and Advanced Generalist Practice';* Vol. 26, 3 (Fall 1990); Wash., D.C. Council of Social Work Education.

Sheafor, Bradford; Horejsi, C. R and Horejsi, G. A. (1988) T*echniques and Guidelines for Social Work Practice*; Boston: Allyn and Bacon, 3rd. ed.

Sontag, Susan (1990) *Illness as Metaphor*; NY; Doubleday.

Thornton, Janet (1937) *The Social Component in Medical Care*; NY; Columbia University Press.

Topliss, Eda (1978) *The Social Context of Health Care*; (eds) Brearly, P; Gibbons, J; Miles A; Topliss, E; Woods, G; Oxford; Basil Blackwood and Mott.

Webster's II New Riverside University Dictionary (1984); NY Houghton Mifflin.

Introduction to the Bio-psychosocial Framework Exemplars

The term 'bio-psychosocial' is both an ecological and a systems one. It is an ecological term in the sense that it implies the processes of *reciprocity* and *mutuality* and the *adaptability* of organism and environment. The term recognises that the environment consists in *levels of social organisation* which are interconnected and have accommodating relationships. It is a systems term in that it implies *linkages* and *interactions* among biological, psychological and social systems which govern human existence. It also implies the systems perspective that changes in one system may effect changes in other systems.

The term 'bio-psychosocial' is often used to imply a holistic approach to human existence that reflects the integration of mind, body and spiritual aspects of the person in a 'whole' sense, as a being who requires balance and harmony in all three dimensions of relationship with himself, the physical and the social environment. The framework also fosters a view of the importance of 'caring' as well as 'curing', an important distinction for health care providers who find they increasingly work with those who can't be 'cured' but who none the less desire to have as good a quality of life as is possible. 'Curing' manifests itself in relation to biological needs. 'Caring' most often manifests itself in relation to psychosocial needs.

The bio-psychosocial framework is an integrative conceptual framework which balances the tendency in medically dominated settings to focus primarily on biological systems. It also serves to remind social workers in medical settings that human beings are as much a biological as a social and psychological creature. The biomedical model of care and existence is a very useful approach to *disease* and has greatly increased our knowledge about its cure and treatment. Physicians are most comfortable with a biomedically definable condition but they are most uncomfortable with ambiguous 'causes' and questionable 'outcomes'. Many physicians are generally uncertain about what can be done to relieve or treat people whose illness is embedded in social environments which they can't influence or control, so they may ignore the social dimensions of health and illness problems.

On the other hand, social workers must usually work on the basis of insufficient data about complex situations, work toward unpredictable outcomes and must often act in the midst of uncertainty. Those oriented to a systems and generalist perspective to social work practice find the bio-psychosocial framework, with its focus on multiple layers of causes and interactions, provides a holistic framework in keeping with the realities of their practice.

Practitioners from all disciplines involved in health care must guard against a lack of appreciation for one dimension of bio-psychosocial understanding at the expense of the other. Social workers must have an appreciation and some understanding of biological systems in order to be useful in the multidisciplinary health care context. They must also be able to speak the language of the biomedical as well as the psychosocial disciplines and be able to help identify interactions between biological systems and social environment factors. Although the bio-psychosocial framework should be the basic concept underlying all social work practice, the following three chapters explore three specific areas of practice in health care where this framework is crucial.

Chapter 2 explores alcohol abuse using the bio-psychosocial perspective. Is alcohol abuse a disease? Is it learnt behaviour that is culturally influenced? What difference does it make to the affected individual, the treatments available, the kind of personnel who provide care or the social policies that govern provision of care? The chapter illustrates the importance, the utilisation and complexities underlying the formal classification systems which social workers must sometimes utilise in multidisciplinary settings. The use of such classification systems have implications for social workers as well as those they serve. The impact of culture on alcohol use and perceptions of alcohol abuse are examined. Chapter 3 focuses on the use of the bio-psychosocial perspective in hospital settings. It reviews the hospital experience and its meaning from the vantage point of the patient and family. It examines the hospital experience from the patient, family and staff perspectives. It details the focus of a psychosocial assessment and its importance for social work practice in medical settings. Chapter 4 focuses on bio-psychosocial aspects of palliative care of cancer patients. It stresses the active total care of patients whose disease is not responsive to curative treatment. Control of pain and of other physical symptoms and of psychological, social and spiritual problems is paramount. The European definition of palliative care stresses that 'illness should not be regarded as an isolated aberration in physiology but considered in terms of the *suffering that it causes the patient and the impact it has on the family*'. Palliative care originated in England but the lessons learnt from hospices world-wide are now being integrated into general medical care. The role of social workers involved in the clinical specialty of oncology provide a model for social workers providing services to other specialised populations facing long term and terminal illness.

Taken together these chapters explore the biological, psychological and social domains of human existence as they manifest themselves in three types of health-related experiences. They examine the levels of intervention, from the personal to the policy level, that may arise from utilising this perspective in relation to health care problems, settings and systems.

References
Cancer Pain Relief and Palliative Care; Report of a World Health Organization Expert Committee; *Technical Report Series* 804; 1990. Geneva; World Health Organization.

Chapter 2
Alcohol Abuse: A Bio-psychosocial Perspective
Beverly Flanigan

This chapter describes alcohol abuse as a social problem with biological, psychological, and social dimensions. It explores similarities and differences between the United States and Russia, the impact of diagnostic and classification systems on treatment, and implications for social work roles and practice.

Similarities and Differences in US and USSR Drinking Practices and Patterns

When comparisons are drawn between the use of alcohol in the United States and the former *Union of Soviet Socialist Republics*, there are a number of similar characteristics. Both countries have had great regional differences in *per capita* consumption of alcohol, probably a reflection of religious and ethnic variations. In the mid-1980s (prior to Gorbachev's anti-drinking campaign), *per capita* alcohol consumption ranged from a high of 14.8 litres in Estonia to a low of 3.44 litres in Azerbaidzhan (Treml, 1991). In the United States in 1984, by comparison, *per capita* consumption ranged from a high of 20.21 litres in Washington, D.C., to a low of 6.35 litres in West Virginia (Williams, Doernberg, Stinson and Noble, 1986). The average *per capita* use was surprisingly similar – 11.8 litres in the USSR and 10.03 litres in the US (Treml, 1991; Williams *et al.*, 1986), although in the past decade, *per capita* consumption in the United States is reported to have steadily decreased (Smith, 1993: *Substance Abuse*).

Another recent similarity between the USSR and the US is the upswing in the numbers of women who drink to excess (Sandmaier, 1980). Some believe there is also an increasing number of young people who are drinking excessively and harmfully. A minority of women and young people probably always drank excessively. However, this is becoming more obvious, in part because of women's entry into the work-force and, in part, because we are learning more about American drinking practices through research.

Important to the discussion of social work's role in the alcoholism field in both countries is the general recognition around the world that a very small proportion of drinkers become 'problem drinkers' or 'alcohol dependent'. The ordinary statistic in the United States is that 9 per cent of drinkers could, at some time, have characteristics describing 'problem drinkers' and/or 'alcoholics' (Akers, 1992; Royce, 1989; Vaillant, 1983). A very similar percentage (10 per cent) is said to be valid in Russia (Anderson and Hibbs, 1992).

In both countries beverage preference also varies from region to region. Among Slavs, vodka and samogon are preferred. In the Baltic states beer is popular, while Moldavians drink more wine (Treml, 1991). By comparison, in 47 of the 50 US states beer is the most-consumed beverage, but there is great variation in the use of spirits and wine. In the southern US states of Mississippi and Arkansas, for example, the *per capita* intake of wine is only 0.41 litres compared with 2.8 litres in California where there are many vineyards and wineries (Williams *et al.*, 1986).[1]

Social Policy Issues
Like other countries, both the United States and the former USSR gather some portion of their taxes from the sales (or manufacturing and distribution) of alcohol. In the USSR in 1985, excise taxes on retail sales, combined with import and production profits, accounted for 13 per cent to 14 per cent of the Soviet's state budget (Treml, 1991). In the United States, the federal government is not involved in production and sales of alcohol, so federal liquor taxes are a far smaller source of federal revenue (0.6 per cent) (United States Bureau of the Census, 1993). However, in states where *per capita* consumption is high, alcohol distributor licences, tavern permits, etc. contribute more to state revenues, but probably not substantially more. It is in countries where tax revenues rely heavily on liquor sales that prohibition against alcohol manufacture and distribution can do great economic damage. The attempt at alcohol prohibition is another shared feature of the United States' and USSR's experience with alcohol.

Prohibition was attempted in the United States between 1920 and 1933 and in Russia between 1914 and 1925 (Fingarette, 1988; Osterberg, 1992; Royce, 1989; Treml, 1991). Both efforts failed. In the United States, prohibition was promoted mostly by middle class Protestants. However, it was unpopular among some newer immigrant and religious groups. While consumption rates did drop, prohibition resulted in increased black market alcohol production and distribution, decreased tax revenues, increased corruption and widespread disregard for regulatory agencies. When prohibition ended, there was a steady return to pre-prohibition consumption rates.

The early Russian prohibition failed for many of the same reasons. Prohibition also failed in Canada, Finland and Norway. When total prohibition fails, most societies with concerns about alcohol consumption then attempt to manipulate the supply-side of alcohol availability. Supply-side manipulation is another common experience of the USSR and the US

The most common approaches to limiting alcohol availability are to manipulate three key policies: the minimum legal drinking age (MLDA), the prices of various beverages, and the sites and business hours of outlets that sell alcoholic beverages. Rationing has been attempted in Sweden and Greenland, but failed for various reasons, particularly the rise of a black market (Osterberg, 1992; Peele, 1987). No country has a single policy that has totally eliminated excessive drinking, but it does appear that the price of alcohol is a potent factor:

> ... a rise in alcohol prices has generally led to a drop in alcohol consumption, and an increase in consumers' income has generally led to a rise in alcohol consumption... Thus, alcoholic beverages appear to behave on the market like other commodities (Osterberg, 1992, 206).

In the USSR, in 1985 the price of vodka doubled and its production was reduced. The result was a dramatic increase in the production and sales of samogon. This, in conjunction with public frustration over long queues, bankrupted vineyards even in regions that drank very little. It caused lost tax revenues, and increased costs of policing needed to combat the sale of 'home brew', ultimately derailing the 1985 anti-drinking campaign (Treml, 1991). Clearly, another common feature of the US and the USSR is that many people in both countries like to drink alcohol!

Supply-side alcohol control efforts are in place in almost every country that has concerns about alcohol use. Their effectiveness is determined by . . . 'social, cultural, and economic characteristics of each country and period [in history]. Therefore each society or state must arrive at its own combination of prevention strategies. . .' (Osterberg, 1992, 210) designed to combat drunkenness, alcohol abuse and alcohol dependency.

Excessive Drinkers: Bad or Sick?

In the United States, there has been a shift over the last fifty years away from viewing the excessive drinker as 'bad', immoral or sinful. Instead, the excessive drinker is viewed as being 'sick' or having the 'disease of alcoholism' (Keller and Doria, 1991; Royce, 1989). This shift has not been as pronounced in the USSR. While there is familiarity with the disease concept in the USSR, people there may view the excessive drinker more as deviant. Therefore, it is appropriate to confine excessive drinkers in the penal system rather than treat them by medical or social services institutions (Anderson and Hibbs, 1992). This point will be detailed later, but it should be noted that, in the US, individuals and their private insurance companies may pay for the treatment of excessive drinking as often as public funds do. Alcoholism, once diagnosed and treated as a disease, can be paid for by insurance companies like any other disease.

Regardless of the paradigmatic view each country may have toward excessive alcohol use, there is no doubt that excessive drinking is connected with adverse social consequences. Alcohol misuse is linked to homicides, driving accidents, violence, crime, rape, domestic violence, and health problems in both countries. In the United States, individual drinking is directly linked to society's perceived social problems. In American culture such 'problems' are to be solved, unlike 'conditions', which are to be tolerated. This distinction between the terms 'problems' and 'conditions' is not an unimportant one. Poor soil, heavy rains, baldness or measles may be conditions that have to be tolerated by countries, communities, families or individuals. Problems, however, such as recurrent crop failure, flooding, or the spread of deadly communicable diseases cannot be tolerated but must be solved.

Excessive drinking in the US is considered a cause of both personal and social problems, so there is the belief that excessive drinking warrants intervention. These interventions may not originate from the penal system but from counsellors, including social workers, who play a crucial role in working with individuals, families and communities. Social workers try to effect change, to help individuals change destructive and self-destructive behaviours that may harm not only themselves and their social groups, but communities and society as well. Social workers also work to change social institutions and policies that may harm individuals. More will be said regarding this later.

Differences Between the USSR and United States Regarding Excessive Alcohol Use

The US and the USSR have uniquely evolved postures toward both alcohol and the people who use it excessively. From our different religious, ethnic, historical, social and political histories, the two countries' differences and similarities have shaped the ways we think about and act toward heavy drinkers. The social work profession in both countries can play a vital role in shaping these thoughts and actions in the future.

Three major differences that prevail between the USSR and United States' views toward excessive alcohol use are important to social workers. These differences are mirrored around the world.

The first is the difference in prevailing philosophies about the nature and causes of excessive use. These differences play themselves out in many ways: (1) in the kinds of professionals who work with alcoholics, (2) the loci of treatment programmes, (3) the kinds of research conducted on excessive alcohol uses, and (4) the kinds of questions asked in the diagnosis of 'alcoholism'.

Alcohol Abuse: A Bio-psychosocial Perspective

The second difference is the emphasis that US researchers and treatment providers place on the effect excessive drinking has on interpersonal relationships, particularly in the drinker's family. In Russia, this emphasis is not widely promoted (Anderson and Hibbs, 1992). In the US, an individual's drunkenness and accompanying behaviour are thought to have profound effects on family members. In fact, negative effects on one's family, when combined with two other symptoms, are enough to warrant a diagnosis of alcohol dependence. Many professionals in the US believe that there do not have to be accidents, problems at work, trouble with the law, drunk driving incidents, crime or other negative social effects of drinking before some interventive action should be taken. If a drinker's family is being physically, psychologically or emotionally hurt, that is enough to warrant intervention (Brown, 1986).

A third difference arises from the prevailing influence of the way prohibitionist thinking, combined with Alcoholics Anonymous, has to some extent stifled creative solutions to alcohol misuse and the way in which alcoholism is both diagnosed and treated. These differences provide opportunities for social workers in both countries to develop creative options for alcohol-dependent people when current approaches to detection or treatment are not effective.

Disparate Philosophies and the Influence of Alcoholics Anonymous
In 1935, Alcoholics Anonymous was established in the US by two men who had been influenced by the thinking of the 'Oxford Group'. This group was an 'evangelically styled attempt to recapture the pietist insight of primitive Christianity' (Kurtz, 1982, 39). The Oxford Group believed in confession of sin, making amends, total honesty, sharing of troubles, and praying to God. The AA founders were also influenced by William James (the 'father of psychology') and his influential work *Varieties of Religious Experience*. Thus, AA sprang from religion and continues to reflect it in 'tone, style, and practice . . .' (Kurtz, 1982, 40).

While AA was taking root, researchers began to examine the men (and not women) who drank to excess. Research tried to identify men's drinking patterns and the character traits that might lead them into drunkenness. The 'disease concept of alcoholism' began to dominate the entire field of alcoholism between 1946 and 1952. It had emerged in the mid-nineteenth century in an era when it became fashionable to 'argue that strange, extreme, or bizarre behaviour and emotional states were caused by mental diseases' (Fingarette, 1988,16). E.M. Jellinek, a researcher, wrote about the experiences of men in AA and how they had become alcoholics. He described their 'progression' into chronic alcoholism. Although he also described other kinds of alcohol misuse patterns, these descriptions generally got lost in the non-scientific community. Jellinek said that in one kind of alcoholism, 'gamma', the drinker lost control of drinking and had withdrawal symptoms if he tried to stop (Jellinek, 1960). In this view, alcoholics were thought to be almost 'allergic' to alcohol. From this point of departure, a virtual flood of research began to examine men who drank.

Meanwhile in the US in the 1930s and 1940s, public inebriates were being jailed or were largely neglected by helping professionals. As a result, alcoholics began to help other alcoholics. Through Alcoholics Anonymous (A.A.), the disease concept of alcoholism began to take hold, even if research failed to entirely endorse it. As in the USSR, sociologists and others (epidemiologists, social workers, psychologists) also began to examine the phenomenon of excessive drinking. Among the hypotheses formulated were that excessive drinking might be: (1) an adaptive reaction to stressors (Cappell, 1987), (2) a symptom of underlying mental health problems, (3) a bad habit (Fingarette, 1988), or (4) an excessive appetite (Orford, 1985). The All-Union Volunteer Temperance Society in the USSR recently 'attacked and succeeded in silencing. . . the group of prominent Soviet sociologists and legal and medical specialists in alcoholism who rejected total abstinence and called for civilised drinking' (Treml, 1991, 130). Likewise some psychologists and sociologists in the United States who view excessive alcohol use as problem drinking that can be changed by behavioural treatment have been sullied professionally and nearly silenced (Pendery, Maltzman and West, 1982).

AA advocates hold to a 'unitary disorder' philosophy of alcoholism. That is, all alcoholism is the same. AA proponents are deeply suspicious of those who believe there may be more than one form or kind of excessive drinking. If excessive alcohol use is a disease, then it can be treated in medical facilities with abstinence as the goal of treatment. If, on the other hand, there are numerous kinds of excessive alcohol use patterns, intervention could come in a variety of forms and delivered by a variety of helping disciplines.

In the United States, the current philosophical sparring in the alcoholism field reflects the exciting, robust intellectual examination of American drinking practices under the scrutiny of disparate disciplines. It also reflects the strong foothold that AA and post-prohibitionist thinking has in the field. However, we currently view excessive alcohol use through so many theoretical lenses that there is a 'lack of consensus on a lexicon in the addiction field [that] impedes communications between professionals of various disciplines, retards deliberation of public policy, and threatens availability of treatment' (Flavin and Morse, 1991, 266).

Alcohol Abuse: A Bio-psychosocial Perspective

Issues in Diagnosis and Classification
The research floodgates having been opened, the 'unitary disorder' promulgated by AA is now giving way to a fuller conceptualisation of excessive alcohol use. Physicians and psychiatrists may continue to search for genetic predeterminants of addictions, sociologists for social conditions that spawn alcohol dependence (such as isolation, homelessness, etc.), and psychologists for personality factors, learning conditions, or expectancies that lead to destructive alcohol use. These efforts are likely to continue to show just how profoundly complex alcohol misuse is.

There are currently two terms that take into account the complexity of excessive alcohol use. The first term designates alcoholism as a 'multivariate syndrome' (Lewis, Dana and Blevins, 1994, 4) and the second designates alcoholism as a 'heterogeneous' (Schuckit, Nathan, Helzer, Woody, and Crowley, 1991) disorder. 'Multivariate syndrome' means that 'drinkers vary in terms of consumption, physical symptoms, patterns of drinking behaviour, life consequences. . ., personality. . ., gender, culture and a variety of other factors' (Lewis *et al.*, 1994, 3). 'Heterogeneous disorder' also means that there are complex causes and patterns of excessive use. Each term acknowledges the complexity of alcohol dependence. The terms do not necessarily indicate, however, the growing acknowledgement of many professionals that since there are many 'causes' and patterns of excessive alcohol use, there may also be many solutions. For example, some solutions may involve alteration of the conditions that contribute to excessive drinking, such as reducing joblessness, homelessness, or stress. Some solutions may involve different ways of providing services to the alcohol-dependent person, such as helping him solve personal problems.

Diagnosis of Alcohol Dependency – Is it Necessary?
A major function of social workers in the alcoholism field in the US is that of assessing and diagnosing alcohol abuse and alcohol dependence. It is a costly and time-consuming endeavour and one that does not necessarily result in differential treatment methods or goals. Traditional treatment, which has dominated the alcoholism field for the past twenty years, does not include individualised treatment goals and methods for different kinds of drinkers. Traditional treatment providers require that all drinkers abstain and counsel only toward abstinence. Therefore, until treatments become more individually tailored, sophisticated differential diagnoses are of little value.

The categories in which social workers and other diagnosticians attempt to place excessive drinkers are (1) 'alcohol dependence' and (2) 'alcohol abuse'. These categories are listed in the official psychiatric *Diagnosis and Statistical Manual of*

Mental Disorders, Third Edition, Revised, 1987 (DSM-IIIR) and the *DSM-IV* (1994), the most widely used and popular diagnostic references for mental health professionals in the United States.

In the *DSM-IIIR,* nine symptoms of alcohol problems are listed. If a person has a score of three or above, and if the symptoms have persisted for a month or more, the individual is labelled *'alcohol dependent'*. The nine symptoms fall under three categories: (1) impaired control, (2) social consequences, and (3) tolerance and withdrawal (American Psychiatric Association, 1987).

A score of two labels a person an *'alcohol abuser'*. A major, if not *the* major, criticism of these criteria is that once a person is diagnosed *'alcohol dependent'* the diagnosis is considered to be a lifelong diagnosis. This implies that the authors of the *DSM-III* and *DSM-IV* 'embody the old cliche... "once an alcoholic, always an alcoholic" — an idea that is not supported by clinical knowledge and empirical findings' (Grant *et al.*, 1991, 291). There is ample evidence in the research that some alcohol-dependent drinkers do drink at some later time in moderation (Akers, 1992; Vaillant, 1983).

Not only does diagnosis in the United States reflect historical and political biases, it is also deeply reflective of European-American prejudices against certain forms of drinking. Different cultures have different views of what constitutes 'normal' and 'abnormal' drinking, but these are not reflected in America's common diagnostic standards.

In Turkey, for example, a normal drinker seeks relaxation and increased sexuality; in Nigeria, relief from stress (Bennett, Janca, Grant and Sartorius, 1992). In the USSR, a normal drinker might see himself as seeking relief from boredom or wanting to have a good time (Treml, 1991).

Abnormal drinking in the United States is thought to begin when: (1) people begin to drink more; (2) spend more time thinking about drinking; (3) experience blackouts and increased tolerance of alcohol; (4) drink more than they intend; (5) have withdrawal symptoms

People with these symptoms are categorised as *'alcohol dependent'*. *'Alcohol abuse'* is purported to exist when a person has recurrent legal or interpersonal problems associated with, or exacerbated by, drinking.

The World Health Organization never had, and does not now have, this kind of classification scheme. Its proposed *International Classification of Diseases – 10th Revision (ICD-10)* classifications include diagnostic categories for the alcohol dependence syndrome and 'the harmful use of alcohol' (Grant *et al.*, 1991, 284).

Alcohol Abuse: A Bio-psychosocial Perspective

The *ICD-10* states that 'the fact that a pattern of use . . . is disapproved or may have led to socially negative consequences, such as arrest or marital arguments is not itself evidence of harmful use . . .': (Jaffe, 1993, 189). In the United States, were these factors present, not only would the label 'alcohol abuse' likely be assigned, but possibly the life-long label of 'alcoholic'. With the *ICD-10* people may be involved in disruptive or illegal behaviour because of the drinking and not be categorised at all.

The distinguishing diagnostic differences between the *DSM-III-R* and *DSM-IV* and the *ICD-10* may seem trivial. However, where professionals have become swept up in the process of diagnosing alcohol dependence so that excessive drinkers can get the services they need, the differences in criteria might result in an individual's being diagnosed as one kind of drinker under one system and quite another kind of drinker in the other. This may have implications for insurance, employability, self-concept and perceived level of deviance in the eyes of family members and the community. Depending on whether there are diverse services available for different kinds of drinkers, professionals in the addiction field in the former USSR and other European countries may decide to spend less time *diagnosing* and more time *treating* people who drink to excess. Social workers in the former USSR, if they diagnose alcohol dependence, will want to choose carefully among the available diagnostic instruments and, perhaps, develop a new one more sensitive to their own cultural drinking norms.

Treatment

Even though the 'unitary concept of alcoholism' is out of step with 'clinical knowledge and empirical findings' (Grant *et al.*, 1991, 291) treatment in the United States is strangely unable to break free from abstinence as the goal of treatment and hospitals or mental health centres as the core of treatment.[2] Abstinence may indeed be a valid treatment objective, but perhaps not the only one; and medical treatment may be an effective method, but again, not the only method of intervention.

Treatment centres in US hospitals generally employ recovering alcoholics, social workers, nurses, and doctors who work in teams to teach people that alcoholism is a disease and that they cannot drink again. Many treatment programmes require people to attend Alcoholics Anonymous. Some programmes bring the family into the programme to help them see that they are not responsible for their family members' alcoholism, that they may carry with them scars that will hurt them later in life or that they may inadvertently set things in motion for the alcoholic to begin drinking again.

In both hospitals and mental health facilities, excessive alcohol users meet together in groups to tell each other about their drinking and to gain support from others in their attempts to quit. Some group and individual treatment programmes, especially for women, focus on previous experiences of physical or sexual abuse that may have precipitated using alcohol as a means of dampening physical and psychological pain. Social workers often lead these groups and teach people about alcohol as a drug and its effects on the body.

Family therapy is an increasingly popular way to intervene in excessive alcohol use. A social worker, as family therapist, might show the family how they use alcohol to avoid each other or to solve problems or to blame one person for the entire family's problems with communication or intimacy (Brolsma, 1986). Some social workers in the US counsel individual drinkers with the presumption that the drinking is symptomatic of other underlying problems such as depression, sociopathy and anxiety. These social workers work in mental health centres or in group practices funded by government fees, client fees, or privately purchased mental health insurance.

While the US has shifted its focus from prohibition to 'treating' the individual problem drinker, it has not formulated an extensive array of sound treatment objectives for the various types of excessive drinkers. The main treatment objective in the United States is 'individual prohibition', even as other countries are introducing many other types of treatment goals. The USSR, by contrast, is using its resources to detect alcoholism and retrain excessive drinkers to learn 'civilised drinking' (Treml, 1991, 125). Both countries could profit from more expansive thinking.

In Russia, where narcologists have traditionally thought of excessive alcohol use as a learnt behaviour that could be unlearnt, the disease concept is being considered more carefully (Anderson and Hibbs, 1992). A blend of the disease/illness model and the learnt behaviour model is now being utilised in many countries (Klingemann *et al.*, 1993), a point that we will return to later. Called the 'alcohol-related problem' approach (Klingemann *et al.*, 1993, 223), this integration of the disease model and the learnt behaviour model offers a variety of treatment methods and goals to fit the individual drinker. USSR social workers may want to promote this more inclusive programme model as they enter the field of addictionology. An inclusive programme model would enable social workers to work with individuals and families on the basis of treatment goals (abstinence or civilised drinking) matched to an individual drinking pattern.

Alcohol Abuse: A Bio-psychosocial Perspective

Social Work Roles: US and the Former USSR
Social workers in the United States engage in the following activities in the alcoholism field. They:

- diagnose alcoholism
- write and promote social policies that drive supply-side manipulation of alcohol availability
- lobby for changes in drunk driving laws and punishments
- work with drivers convicted of drunk driving to teach them about alcohol
- counsel excessive drinkers
- do out-patient group work
- administer and staff detoxification centres
- work in industry to refer workers whose drinking causes problems with productivity
- develop and run community and school preventive education programmme
- counsel family members of alcoholics
- set up and run 'half-way' houses where people who are trying to stop drinking live together for temporary support
- develop programmes for communities to make available new recreational activities where drinking is not allowed (these programmes are often developed for young people)
- work with people leaving penal institutions to warn them of the dangers of excessive drinking, and
- work with homeless people who drink excessively to assist them to find food, shelter and clothing, and at the same time to stop drinking.

Social workers in the United States may be employed to provide services in hospitals, mental health centres, schools, industries, detoxification centres, homeless shelters, half-way houses, community centres, community support programmes and state government agencies.

The remainder of this chapter will explore how social workers might be used in the wisest way in the field of narcology. To some extent, evolutionary developments in the United States have helped shape social workers' functions as much as strategic planning. Social workers in the former Soviet Union might borrow from US social workers' experiences, but tailor the US experience to their own culture and the evolutionary developments of social work as a profession in their own countries.

If social workers in the former USSR could create their own involvement in narcology, they might first convene groups to meet together to decide which social work functions are necessary, which social work functions are possible, and which functions are feasible for social workers to do. But first, social workers should decide which problems created by excessive drinking they will choose to devote their energies and resources to resolving.

There are four critical problem areas that social workers address in the field of alcoholism: (1) family problems, (2) health problems, (3) mental health problems, and (4) social problems such as violence, rape, homicides, public misbehaviour. Research shows that, where family problems are concerned, children of alcoholics may have more behaviour problems than children of non-alcoholics (Jacob and Leonard, 1986). These children may also become alcoholics more often than other people (Brown, 1986). Also noted is the finding that spouses of alcoholics who have fewer emotional problems than spouses who have more extensive mental health problems, are less likely to have children who are damaged by alcoholism (Jacob and Leonard, 1986). In the area of health, life-expectancy in Russia is said to be decreasing because of extensive drinking (Treml, 1991). It is widely known that excessive alcohol use can also do damage to the heart (Smith, 1986), liver (Lieber, 1976), and bones (Diamond, Stiel, Lunzer, Wilkerson and Posen, 1989) and is linked with numerous cancers (Hoffman and Heinemann, 1986). Excessive drinking is also associated with foetal damage and Foetal Alcohol Syndrome (Aase, 1994). Regarding mental health, excessive use is tied to depression and some personality disorders. Certainly there is a link between alcohol dependence and many social problems such as domestic violence, automobile accidents, and homicides. Figure 1 indicates the four problem areas, potential social work methods, and possible sites in which social workers might intervene.

Alcohol Abuse: A Bio-psychosocial Perspective

Figure I

Type of Problem	Social Work Method	Service Site
Family problems	Counselling alcoholic and family	In homes of alcoholic At sobering-up stations Medical or mental health centres
	Teaching children	Community centres Schools
	Counselling spouses of alcoholics in groups Teaching communities about drinking	Community Centres Town/village meetings
Mental health problems	Diagnosing and referring	
	Counselling alcoholics in groups	Mental health/hospital/ industrial settings People's home, work places
Social problems	Creating new recreational opportunities	Community councils/centres Church groups
	Developing new local policies for requiring alcoholics who damage the community to make restitution	Community councils Community leaders convene in groups
	Developing new recreational, learning spiritual resource	Neighbourhoods, small groups of families working together
Health problems	Teaching people about adverse effects of alcohol: liver damage, foetal damage, etc.	Schools - Industries Market places Newspapers - Television
	Helping to manage alcohol-related health problems as member of interdisciplinary teams	Hospitals and clinics

Figure 1 suggests that if social workers decide, for example, that excessive alcohol use affects families in more critical ways than it affects mental health, physical health, or society, then the profession might offer counselling and education in the service site suggested. Social workers could work in schools, homes, community centres or medical centres and polyclinics. Counsellors could (1) help family members understand that they are not responsible for another person's excessive alcohol use; (2) help families decide how to carry on together if the drinker insists on excessive use (that is, help children and spouses learn how to defend themselves against verbal and physical abuse and find ways to form a healthy family life regardless of alcohol misuse); or (3) provide support to family members if the family breaks up.

If social workers decide to tackle mental health problems of alcohol-dependent people (Figure 1), they could work in hospitals, industries, and health/mental health facilities. Their work could include problem identification, counselling, and helping people work together to create recreational or spiritual opportunities that do not include drinking. Counselling would involve (1) helping drinkers determine the reasons they drink excessively; (2) helping drinkers to determine specific goals such as reduction in drinking, alteration of the contexts of drinking, or total abstinence; and (3) providing cognitive and behavioural tools to help the drinker meet his goals. Social workers could also counsel alcohol-dependent people in groups so that group members learn how to support each other in reaching their drinking-reduction and other life goals.

Figure 1 also indicates where social workers might find a place in helping to alleviate social problems and health problems associated with alcohol abuse. Given that in all probability social workers cannot address all forms of these problem areas equally, it follows that the profession must place its resources where the problems are most critical. Most likely health and family problems are especially important because they affect the future of children in very direct ways.

Finally, social workers in the former Soviet Union may choose to advocate for a model of intervening in alcohol abuse that is holistic and all-encompassing. If the service sites suggested in Figure 1 do not now exist, alcohol-specific agencies might be developed. In these decentralised centres, social workers could take referrals, teach, diagnose, counsel and refer clients to outside resources if further help is needed. Research could also be conducted there. All-purpose agencies that recognise alcohol abuse as having many causes, symptoms, and solutions are becoming more common throughout the world.

It seems not only that many countries have switched from a 'moral' model of alcoholism to an 'illness' model but also that the concept of alcoholism as a disease is being replaced by that of 'alcohol-related problems' (Morawski, 1992, in Klingemann *et al.*, 222-223).

Poland's treatment system uses the moral, illness, and alcohol-related problems models together. New Zealand, Switzerland, the UK and Sweden apparently do the same.

Summary

Social work, as a new profession in many countries of the former USSR, has a rare opportunity to create its own mission. Given that attempts at limiting drinking through outright prohibition have not succeeded, some experts believe that resources should be directed toward that 10 per cent of drinkers who have, and are likely to cause, problems (Anderson and Hibbs, 1992). These drinkers are at high risk for health and mental health problems, and their children might learn or inherit these problems as well. Social work across the world reaches out to groups at risk — to prevent, diagnose, treat and counsel in light of their special needs. Social workers in the former USSR have a unique opportunity to contribute their ideas to what diagnostic method might be selected for identifying alcohol-dependent people. Social workers can recommend that various kinds of drinkers are provided various kinds of treatment objectives. Social workers can establish programmes for families and children living with an alcohol-dependent person so that the damage of alcohol abuse is contained. Social workers can design and teach (or train others to teach) about drinking and the effects of alcohol on pregnancy, driving, industrial accidents and damage to physical organs such as the heart and kidney.

Problems should not be feared by social work. Instead, they should be recognised, analysed, and taken on in order to develop creative solutions. Social workers, applying their unique 'problem-solving perspective', are poised to make significant contributions to the problems of individuals and society. Alcohol abuse, affecting both, should be a priority of the new social work profession as it emerges in countries of the former Soviet Union — a priority that generates creative, humane services for alcohol abusers, their families, and their communities.

Notes

1. Both denizens of the former USSR and Americans may be surprised to learn that in the United States, the *per capita* consumption during the late 1700s and 1800s was probably twice as high as it is today. Spread evenly among men, women and children *per capita* consumption was roughly 15 litres per person

(Fingarette, 1988). Today, a small proportion of drinkers (around 11 per cent) drink roughly 55 per cent of all the alcohol consumed.

2. There is much to be said about the success rates of treatment programmes. However, this is beyond the scope of this paper. Overall, roughly two out of three people who have been treated with abstinence as their goals have drunk again after treatment (Vaillant, 1983).

References

Aase, J.M. (1994) *Clinical recognition of FAS, Alcohol Health and Research World*, 18(1), 5-9.

Akers, R.L. (1992). *Drugs, Alcohol and Society*. Wadsworth, Belmont.

American Psychiatric Association (1987). *Diagnostic and Statistical Manual of Mental Disorders, 3rd Edition, Revised (DSM-III-R)*, The Association, Washington, D.C.

Anderson, S.C., and Hibbs, V.K. (1992). Alcoholism in the Soviet Union, *International Social Work*, 35, 441-453.

Bennett, L.A., Janca, A., Grant, B.F., and Sartorius, N. (1992). Boundaries between normal and pathological drinking, *Alcohol Health and Research World*, 17(3), 190-196.

Beresford, T.P. (1991). The nosology of alcoholism research, *Alcohol Health and Research World*, 15(4), 260-265.

Brolsma, J.K. (1986). Family therapy in the treatment of alcoholism. In N.J. Estes and M.E. Heinemann (eds) *Alcoholism Development, Consequences and Interventions*, Mosby, St Louis.

Brown, S. (1986). Children with an alcoholic parent. In N.J. Estes and M.E. Heinemann (eds) *Alcoholism Development, Consequences and Interventions*, Mosby, St Louis.

Cappell, H. (1987). Alcohol and tension reduction: What's new? In E. Gottheil (ed.) *Stress and Addiction*, Brunner/Mazel, New York.

Diamond, T., Stiel, D., Lunzer, M., Wilkerson, M., and Posen, S. (1989). Ethanol reduces bone formation and may cause osteoporosis, *American Journal of Medicine*, 86(3), 282-288.

Fingarette, H. (1988). *Heavy Drinking*, University of California Press, Berkeley.

Flavin, D.K., and Morse, R.M. (1991). What is alcoholism?, *Alcohol Health and Research World*, 15(4), 266-271.

Grant, B.F., and Towle, L.H. (1991). A comparison of diagnostic criteria,*Alcohol Health and Research World*, 15(4), 284-292.

Hoffman, A.C., and Heinemann, M.E. (1986). Alcohol problems in elderly persons. In N.J. Estes and M.E. Heinemann (eds) *Alcoholism Development, Consequences and Interventions,* Mosby, St Louis.

Jacob, T., and Leonard, L. (1986). Psychosocial functioning in children of alcoholic fathers, depressed fathers and control fathers, *Journal of Studies on Alcohol*, 47(5), 373-380.

Jaffe, J.H. (1993). The concept of dependence, *Alcohol Health and Research World*, 17(3), 188-189.

Jellinek, E.M. (1960). *The Disease Concept of Alcoholism*, Hillhouse Press, Highland Park.

Keller, M., and Doria, J. (1991). On defining alcoholism, *Alcohol Health and Research World*, 15(4), 253-259.

Klingemann, H., Takala, J., and Hunt, G. (1993). The development of alcohol treatment systems. *Alcohol Health and Research,* 17(3), 221-227.

Kurtz, E. (1982). Why AA works, *Journal of Studies on Alcohol,* 43(1), 38-80.

Lewis, J.A., Dana, R.Q., and Blevins, G.A. (1994). *Substance Abuse Counselling*, 2nd Edition, Brooks/Cole, Pacific Grove.

Lieber, C.S. (1976). The metabolism of Alcohol, *Scientific American*, 234, 25-38.

Orford, J. (1985). *Excessive Appetites: A Psychological View of Addictions,* Wiley, New York.

Osterberg, E. (1992). Global status of alcohol control research, *Alcohol Health and Research World*, 17(3), 205-211.

Peele, A. (1987). The limitations of control-of-supply models for explaining and preventing alcoholism and drug addiction, *Journal of Studies on Alcohol*, 48, 61-77.

Pendery, M., Maltzman, I.M., and West, L.J. (1982). Controlled drinking by alcoholics: New findings and a reevaluation of a major affirmative study, *Science*, 217, 169-175.

Royce, J.E. (1989). *Alcohol Problems and Alcoholism*, Free Press, New York.

Sandmaier, M. (1980). *The Invisible Alcoholic: Women and Alcohol Abuse in America*, McGraw-Hill, New York.

Schuckit, M.A., Nathan, P.E., Helzer, J.E., Woody, G.E., and Crowley, T.J. (1991). Evolution of the DSM Diagnostic Criteria for Alcoholism, *Alcohol Health and Research World*, 15(4), 278-292.

Selzer, M.L. (1971). The Michigan Alcoholism Screening Test (MAST): The quest for a new diagnostic instrument, *American Journal of Psychiatry*, 3, 176-181.

Smith, J.W. (1986) Alcohol and disorders of the heart and skeletal muscles. In N.J. Estes and M.E. Heinemann (eds) *Alcoholism Development, Consequences and Interventions*, Mosby, St Louis.

(1993). *Substance Abuse: The Nation's Number One Health Problem. Institute for Health Policy*, Brandeis University, Robert Wood Johnson Foundation, Princeton.

Treml, V.G. (1991). Drinking and alcohol abuse in the USSR in the 1980s. In A. Jones, W.D. Connor, and D. Powell (eds) *Soviet Social Problems*, Westview Press, Boulder.

United States Bureau of the Census (1993). *Statistical Abstracts of the United States*, Government Printing Office, Washington, D.C.

Vaillant, G.E. (1983). *The Natural History of Alcoholism*, Harvard University Press, Cambridge.

Williams, G., Doernberg, D., Stinson, F., and Noble, J. (1986). State, regional and national trends in apparent *per capita* consumption. *Alcohol Health and Research World*, 10(4), 60-63.11.

Chapter 3
Social Work Practice in Hospital Settings: A Bio-psychosocial Perspective
Norma Berkowitz

Introduction
An essential objective of social work practice in health care is the development, maintenance or restoration of 'personhood' to those who are ill or disabled. Social workers in hospitals face this challenge in a unique setting, in an institution dominated by an ethos and approach to the human condition which is quite different from that of social work. This chapter presents a context for social work practice in hospital settings and explores, briefly, basic themes and concepts.

The Hospital Experience: A Patient's View
The Patient's 'Work'

Hospitals share some of the qualities of total institutions: those who enter them as patients would, all things considered, rather not have to enter them. Once they enter, they are not at liberty to leave them at will. Cast in the role of 'patient' the person even in the most humane hospital with the most sensitive staff runs the risk of becoming dehumanised, seen as an object to be viewed, manipulated and treated. For example, staff often use shorthand phrases to refer to a patient as the 'cancer' in bed 134 or the 'stroke' in ward 3.

The concept of the 'patient role' derives from the general concept of role theory that emerged from sociology in the 1950s. By virtue of entry into the hospital, an individual changes role status. Instead of the role of independent, autonomously functioning individual, a person is assigned the new role of 'patient'. Patients lose the right to determine their daily schedule of activities and become dependent on those who presumably have the power to heal or cure them. This engenders feelings of hopelessness and lack of control over one's life which in turn often stimulates feelings of depression or anger.

Organisational barriers, short stays and high patient turnover also prevent development of a sense of 'community' in hospital settings. There is no way for patients to learn from others the rules and norms governing their new role status. The situation is compounded when the hospital is short of staff and over-worked personnel do not have the time to provide information, personal comfort and social support to individual patients.

The patients are also faced with a variety of tasks which they are implicitly or explicitly expected to accomplish. Many of these are self-care tasks (such as bathing, toileting and eating). Staff expect patients to carry out these tasks to the maximum extent possible. Patients are also expected to provide careful and accurate data during interviews. They are expected to accurately report discomforts and levels of pain. Demands are made of them during various tests: 'make a fist', 'tell me when it hurts', 'ring the buzzer when the bag is empty', 'work the treadmill until you feel you can't possibly go any longer', etc.

Patients also become students; in effect they may be educated about how to monitor the machines they are hooked up to, how to administer their own pain medication, or how to attach orthopaedic devices. These expectations have an effect on patient behaviour because in light of such expectations they hesitate to complain, they fear failure to comply, and they may not provide adequate feedback, especially to nurses and doctors. This, in turn, may impede the patient's progress toward recovery.

The patient may also be involved in tasks which require expenditures of effort, resolve and courage, such as when a person is in severe pain and must change body position, or must drink medicine which is distasteful, or take a deep breath when it hurts. There are often embarrassing tasks associated with bodily functions, such as producing urine, faeces or sputum on demand.

Patient and Staff Relationships

All of this requires co-operation with staff (Tagliacozzo and Mauksch, 1988). Should patients refuse, or be unable to comply, they are frequently cajoled, teased, or scolded. This further demeans the patient and contributes to lowered self-esteem. It reduces the motivation needed to successfully engage with hospital staff and accomplish the medical regimen needed for successful treatment outcomes.

Hospital staff members generally expect patients to be co-operative so treatments will proceed smoothly. Some staff members have been trained to teach, encourage and support patients in ways which help patients accomplish their tasks. Other staff, however, may quickly label a patient 'non-compliant', 'stubborn', 'inconsiderate', or 'obstinate', thus compounding the debilitating effects on the patient.

These dynamics of role behaviours on the part of both staff and patient are a key focus of social workers operating in a professional capacity in a hospital setting and are a legitimate target for social work intervention. Sometimes negative behaviours on the part of staff impede patient progress and sometimes negative behaviours on the part of the patient and/or attitudes and behaviours of family members impinge on patients' relations with staff.

Regardless of the source, negative feelings and behaviours invariably impede a patient's progress and prolong hospitalisation. This is especially true of the doctor-patient relationship. There is an increasing body of research indicating that the way a doctor is perceived by patients often determines if they follow directions (compliance) and how quickly they recover. In a sample of patients following life-threatening recovery, 'style of doctoring' affected speed of recovery (Auberach, 1989). In a survey of 300 former patients of a community hospital, 99 per cent of the respondents felt the most important aspect of quality hospital care was getting an explanation from their doctors of what was going to happen to them. Attentiveness of doctors and responsiveness of nurses and other staff to patient needs were ranked second by 97 per cent of respondents (Meyer & Abubaker, 1988). Criticisms of patient relationships with doctors have to do with poor communication, depersonalisation, not spending sufficient time with patients and families. Some of the same criticisms apply to patient/nurse relationships, partly due to the perception of the nurse as being overworked and wielding considerable power over the life of a temporarily dependent patient. In light of this, as part of programme evaluation, many hospital social work departments are now conducting 'patient satisfaction surveys' which generally indicate positive results of patient/social work relations.

The relationship between social worker, patient and physician is critical for achieving the agenda for social work in hospital settings. This agenda is to influence patient care, to make it more responsive to patient needs so the patient may engage successfully with a treatment regimen and reap its benefits, and to minimise the pain and suffering of the patient. This agenda can only be accomplished if the social worker establishes positive relationships with the physicians with whom they work.

Relationships with physicians should have the common elements and characteristics of all social work relationships. *They are formed for a professional purpose, are devoted to the interests of clients, not self-interest, are based on objectivity and self-awareness*, allowing the social worker to step outside personal needs and be sensitive to the needs of another. Relationships with physicians, nurses and patients can be conflictual, bargaining, collegial and/or political. They involve consensus-building strategies, negotiating strategies, coalition building and conflict resolution strategies. Nearly always, social workers gain acceptance in medical settings when: (1) they are seen to be competent and successful in implementing patient and physician objectives; (2) they become valued as a provider of concrete services (such as finding homecare resources, financial assistance or transportation services); (3) are perceived as accurate in the observation and recording of needed data; (4) make special contributions in cases where psychosocial and cultural problems complicate medical care; (5) are dependable and trustworthy; and (6) function as empathic colleagues.

The quality of staff/patient interactions may be affected by such things as the sex, education and socio-economic level, and previous hospital experience, of patients. The interactions may also be affected by the sex, education and socio-economic status, the in-service training of the staff, and the level of staffing in the hospital. Cultural background and health beliefs of both patients and staff also influence these interactions.

The Existential Task
In addition to the tasks staff expect of them, patients must also learn to cope with existential questions such as: 'Why is this happening to me? Who am I? How will this change my life?' Because the task of coping is not observable, many staff undervalue or ignore the importance of it. However, these questions represent a threat to 'personhood' that drains a patient's strength and energy and opens the possibility of a world that doesn't operate according to the principle of 'fairness'. This can pose a threat to the metaphysical belief system which has governed the patient's life prior to the onset of illness and/or hospitalisation.

Coping with these questions involves motivation, cognition, problem-solving abilities, planning and judgement, self-esteem and self-confidence, and utilising defences against anxiety and depression. Coping strategies are directed (1) to preserving a reasonable emotional balance, (2) to preserving a satisfactory self-image, (3) to preserving relationships with family and friends and (4) to preparing for an uncertain future (Moos and Tsu, 1977).

Attention to suffering that may be engendered by these existential questions is considered one of the primary ends of medicine by patients and lay persons. However, many members of the medical profession perceive the relief of pain but not the relief of existential suffering as their mission.

Based on clinical observations Cassel makes a distinction between suffering and physical distress such as pain. Suffering can INCLUDE physical pain but is by no means LIMITED to it. Suffering is experienced by persons, not merely by bodies. Suffering has as its source the challenges that threaten the intactness of the person as a complex social and psychological, as well as a biological, entity (Cassell, 1982).

Social Work Practice in Hospital Settings: A Bio-psychosocial Perspective

Social workers in hospitals, drawing on their humanistic value base, tolerance for a diversity of cultural backgrounds, and a framework described as bio-psychosocial, are in a position to help patients address the existential crises and suffering which may be precipitated by admission to hospital. Often patients deal with such crises by relying on spiritual understanding or religious beliefs which differ from those of the physician or nurses caring for them. However, hospital staff must respect cultural and religious beliefs in order to facilitate the patient's impetus toward understanding and coping with issues of personhood and existential meaning (Turner and Mapa, 1988).

When assessing coping styles and skills, coping is viewed as a process-over-time and it is only as a person's illness progresses that a social worker can judge the adaptive potential of a patient's or family's particular coping strategies.

The Hospital Experience: A Family Perspective
Hospital entry catapults both patients and family members into a complex social system with its own rules, traditions and culture. This world is alien and intimidating to most families, especially since those entering the system frequently know nothing about its norms and expectations. Family members also feel they lack the skills needed to accomplish the tasks expected of them. They may feel totally helpless due to lack of information and feelings of uncertainty about the future course of the hospitalisation. They are intimidated by hospital language, technology and routines.

Just as the patient is cast in the role of 'patient', families are cast in the role of 'patient's family'. In this role, families also are expected to be co-operative, not be too demanding of hospital staff, not interfere with treatment procedures, obey the scheduled visiting hours and any restrictions on providing comfort care to the patient.

Family members and kin are not given an explicit part to play in patient care. However, three types of 'kin work' have been identified (Strauss,1984):

(1) Working with a patient 'psychologically'. This often involves: (a) offering reassurance and encouragement; (b) being a physical presence which offers physical comfort, for example arranging pillows and (c) being a social presence which offers social support by retaining connections with 'home'; (d) sharing feelings and ideas about life and death, joint exploration of questions such as 'why did this happen to me?'; (e) sharing recollections and memories of past life; (f) helping the patient explicitly express levels of pain and discomfort;

(g) providing opportunities for patients to discuss unfinished business such as past injuries they've caused or experienced, or to ask forgiveness of someone against whom they have transgressed.

(2) Families often do legal-administrative work on behalf of the patient. When a patient is unable to give permission or sign certain documents, bureaucratic problems may result. Certain kin in certain situations may act as a patient's agent to minimise consequences of bureaucratic problems. Kin may perform such tasks as notifying appropriate insurance agencies, preparing documents or agreements necessary for distribution of property, gain information for death records or make funeral arrangements. The greater the bureaucratisation of hospital services and the higher the degree of technological care provided, the more important this becomes. Family members also may become advocates for the patient by making the patient's needs and wishes known to the staff.

(3) Families often engage the patient in crucial decision-making. Kin support and participation with the patient on the work that needs to be done in the course of hospitalisation help overcome fear, anxiety and loneliness. Kin participation also provides the arena in which patients can review situations requiring decision-making and explore options in the knowledge that family members best know their psychological make up, their life experience and their social situation.

When family members are unaware of ways they may be helpful to patients, social workers may sensitise them to the patient's needs and help them learn how to help their family member cope with the hospitalisation and illness process. By helping family members provide social support to the patient, social workers increase the social resources available to the patient to help deal with the illness experience.
If no family members assume these responsibilities, the social worker often assumes them as part of the professional task.

Crisis Intervention
When hospitalisation is the result of an unexpected acute illness or trauma, or an unexpected development during the course of an otherwise chronic illness, this represents an additional crisis to the patient and family. A crisis may also be precipitated by unexpected news that surgery will be required or that an illness is terminal, or that death is imminent. In these situations some people react by perceiving the illness event as so dangerous that they are unable to cope effectively.

Crisis intervention is another major focus of social work practice in hospital settings. Originally crisis theory was rooted in psychoanalytic personality theory and preventive psychiatry. Its modern formulation is a synthesis of systems concepts, ego psychology, stress theory, existentialism and learning theory. This synthesis emphasises how the human system adapts to stressors in a way that new growth and learning can occur. The theory extends and enriches the concept of the person: situation configuration as the unit of attention in psychosocial intervention.

The goal of crisis intervention is to alleviate the immediate impact of disruptive stressful events that threaten life, security, and/or relationships of individuals involved. This is accomplished by mobilising the psychological strengths and social resources of those directly affected by the situation or event.

Crisis intervention is an approach to providing assistance that is characterised by (1) being immediately available, (2) focusing primarily on alleviating stress, (3) minimally interfering with the individual's usual patterns of being and coping, and (4) providing increasing therapeutic intervention as needed. It is an appropriate initial intervention in many situations because it may help people (a) partialise rather than globalise the crisis, (b) reduce tension, (c) realistically appraise the dangerousness of the situation, (d) stimulate cognitive awareness and emotional significance of the situation, and (e) help identify ways of beginning to cope with it (Golan, 1978).

The experience of crisis precipitated by hospitalisation is perceived differently by the patient and by the family. The patient experiences this crisis as a threat to personhood and to continued physical existence. The family experiences it as a threat to the possible loss of a loved one and a loss that will precipitate changes in the role structure of the family. Both may be overwhelmed by the unexpectedness of the situation, lack of information, the strangeness and complexity of the hospital setting, disruption of everyday life (such as employment, parenting role, and responsibilities for care of other family members). Therefore, crisis intervention strategies can legitimately be directed to both patients and their families.

In crisis intervention, social workers must (1) do rapid assessments of both patient's and family's needs, (2) direct intervention toward focused goals identified by patient or family, (3) work toward solutions of current problems and (4) work with patient and family members as collaborators in the problem-solving process.

Effective use of crisis intervention strategies helps patients and families to cope, to manage stress as successfully as possible. Coping is the active, conscious process of dealing with stress, as compared with the use of unconscious defence mechanisms which are more integrated into personality structure. As already noted, coping is successful when it helps avoid or reduce feelings of stress, reduces the number of, or severity of presenting, problems, and maintains a positive sense of self.

Family as the Basic Unit of Focus
In the United States the important link between patient and family during hospitalisation is in keeping with a primary shift in social work away from viewing the individual as the basic unit of concern and casework as the primary intervention. It is important in health care situations to view the family as the basic unit of health management, health education and practices. Family members are also often care givers. A family approach is crucial in dealing effectively with the health care and concerns of the patient. This focus complements a systems framework as a basic theoretical orientation for social work practice, a framework which understands the world in terms of relatedness, transactions and synthesis.

Family centred practice is a model of social work practice which locates the family in the centre of attention or the field of action (Germain, 1980) and defines what social work attends to (Meyer 1976). It draws heavily on the experience of therapists utilising concepts evolved from a variety of systems approaches and strategies used in family therapy.

As a model for social work, family centred practice has as its focus those transactions among person, family and environment which affect individuals, families and even the larger social forces and systems in which they are enmeshed. (Hartman and Laird, 1983). Changes in life expectancy, changes in family structure due to divorce and single parenting, changes in family roles as more women work full time — all affect family functioning.

Hospitalisation or the advent of a chronic illness impacts heavily on family functioning and multi-generational concerns which must be explored as part of social work practice in hospital and clinic settings.

Perspectives on Social Work in Hospital Settings
Historically, social work practice in health care in the United States has been associated with the term 'medical social work'. It began in the early 1900s with the training of social workers to work in hospital settings.

In the health care contexture the term '*clinical social work*' has replaced the older concept of '*medical social work*'. This term describes the practice of social work with, and on behalf of, patients. It includes collaborative activities between social workers and members of the medical and paramedical professions. It includes the full range of activities reflected in the social work process in health care and permits a range of interventions and methods as prescribed by generalist practice (Carlton, 1984).

Social Work Practice in Hospital Settings: A Bio-psychosocial Perspective

This clinically oriented social work practice in hospital settings is rooted in the basic orientation, history, value base and process common to all social work practice. It reflects a *professional*, rather than a *technical* orientation. It focuses on social interactions and person:environment exchanges and adaptations. However, because the context in which professional practice occurs is not the *social service system* but the *medical service system*, there are unique aspects to practice in hospitals.

Hospitals are designated as the place where people with disease and life-threatening disabilities go for cure and/or treatment in order to sustain or extend life. The primary focus is on disease, the actual deterioration of an organ by invasion from a destructive agent (for example bacteria or viruses).

The primary focus of hospital social work is that of attending to the WHOLE of the patient's human existence and promulgating the view of the patient as a *psychological* and *social* being as well as a physical being. Social workers in medical settings must guard against the dualism of the medical profession which tends toward the separation of 'mind' and 'body' proposed by the philosopher Decartes; a concept that has deeply influenced approaches to modern medical care.

However, a major shift in this concept of dualism is occurring as the result of a growing body of research findings in cognitive psychology and in biomedical research. This research indicates that immune system functioning may be affected by cognitions and thoughts which in turn affect mood, which in turn may affect the activity of the brains neurotransmitters and a cell's vulnerability to attack by viruses. Some of these interactions are now visible using sophisticated computer technology.

Multidisciplinary Teams
Social workers in hospital settings also work in a context which demands continuous contact with members of other disciplines and professions. These relationships must be positive ones if social work interventions are to be effective in bettering the situation of the patient and fostering an atmosphere in which the patient's needs may be met. This close alliance often requires working in multidisciplinary teams. In hospitals in which there are no designated teams, it is none the less necessary to effectively participate in what has been identified as 'collaborative practice' (Dana, 1983).

Dana accepts 'the need to work in tandem with other professions and disciplines as a basic requirement for social work's effectiveness as an instrumentality of health and medical care' (Dana, l983). Carlton points out that 'interdisciplinary' is another term used for describing various forms of collaborative practice in social work. Such collaboration is defined as 'interdisciplinary practice by two or more practitioners from two or more fields of learning and activity, who fill distinct roles, perform specialised tasks and work in an interdependent relationship toward the achievement of a common purpose' (Carlton, 1984). Both these writers recognise the need for social workers to be firmly grounded in the values, knowledge and skills of social work practice before they can be an effective participant in the collaborative process.

Collaboration in health care is concerned with the sick and disabled, wherever they are encountered, and rests on: (1) recognition of the interplay of psychological, social and biological factors in the cause, course and outcome of disease; (2) recognition of the strength and power of the multiple forces that support a holistic approach to human problems; (3) the need to keep humanism alive as a condition of the human services (Dana, 1983).

The ability to engage successfully in collaborative practice demands special attitudes and cognitive attributes of the professional. The stance in collaborative practice is one of *interdependence rather than either independence or dependence*. This stance is rooted in a strong identity as a social worker but at the same time the social worker 'recognises and accepts the fact that members of other health professions and disciplines not only have unique knowledge and skills to bring to the study and solution of health problems but also have legitimate claims to the caring and coping functions which are too often viewed as the private domain of social work' (Dana, 1983).

Historically, there have been strains in the social workers' relationship with both physicians and nurses. While this strain is generally attributed to 'the medical model' or 'disease' orientation of medical care, five conflicting values of the professions may interfere with their ability to work collaboratively: (1) attitudes toward saving life versus quality of life; (2) attitudes toward patient autonomy in setting treatment goals; (3) attitudes toward the use of objective versus subjective data; (4) differential responses to patients with emotional problems; (5) differing perspectives on interdisciplinary team roles (Roberts, 1989).

Besides value differences between the various disciplines represented on multi-disciplinary teams in hospitals, struggles for turf, power and control are major obstacles to collaborative practice. The extent to which these become manifest are often due to personality attributes of the team members, for example the degree to which their self-esteem is threatened by loss of control or power. Thus not only the perception of professional expertise, but the behavioural components of respect and honesty, openness, communication style, and general 'liking' of the social worker by other members of the team have direct influence on how effectively the social worker's information and recommendations are utilised.

Astute social workers recognise that many of the principles involved in establishing and maintaining sound relationships with clients are applicable to working with colleagues from other disciplines. Empathy and respect for others' positions and contributions are critical.

Colleagues from other disciplines often must be taught about the contributions social workers make to the well-being of patients and families by engaging in joint problem solving. The contributions social workers make to the collaborative team also need to be learnt. One contribution social workers make is to help the team deal with the emotional environment surrounding the collaborative process. This process inevitably engenders the need to deal with competitive feelings and with authority, shared disappointments when things go wrong and shared elation when things work out, domination or power issues posed by a team member, and valid professional differences of opinion.

Another influence on effective collaboration is the level of knowledge participants have about group dynamics and group process. Social workers knowledgeable and experienced in group process often identify for teams, or others involved in a collaborative process, the characteristics of the developmental stage through which participants are passing. Dana identifies stages in the collaborative 'learning through doing' process as: the becoming acquainted stage, the trial and error stage, the collective indecision stage, the crisis stage and the resolution stage (Dana, 1983). Helping teams and/or those involved in the collaborative process identify emotional aspects or developmental phases in team process helps members cope with problem-solving tasks.[1]

The Clinical Social Work Process in Hospital Settings

Acceptance of social work practice as a problem-solving process focuses attention on person, problem, place, process, the client:worker relationship and mutually-agreed-upon problem-solving work. This process is the same in hospital settings as in other social work practice settings and is based on the same values. The process involves: (1) developing an agreed statement of the problem; (2) the identification of causal factors; (3) development of a plan of action (which includes identification of needs, determination of objectives and selection of intervention procedures and tasks); and (4) provisions for termination, evaluation and feedback. The process is client focused but the degree to which the hospital patient is permitted to function autonomously is deterred by having acquired 'patient status'.

The social worker's task is to engage the client in a process of problem solving that maximises opportunities for client control and decision making even though this often involves: (1) balancing risks against safety, (2) choices among less than perfect solutions, and (3) recognising restraints due to economic, social, or legal considerations or lack of personal and community resources.

In the light of the medical personnel's commitment to the biological aspects of a patient's well-being, a special part of the social work process in hospital settings focuses on assessing the influence that psycho-social factors play in the patient's condition, how these factors might affect the trajectory of the illness or the hospital stay, and the role these factors might play in the recovery or rehabilitation process. Ability to assess the *social dimensions of a particular patient's situation* is as important as others' ability to diagnose the biological and psychological dimensions of patient care since often the social element can be directly or indirectly as life threatening as the physical illness or its psychological impact.

Psychosocial Assessment

The 'psychosocial' dimension implies an interactive process between the inner psychological processes of an individual as they affect or are affected by, the outer components of experience, the environment. Psychosocial assessment attempts to clarify this relationship between inner psychological processes and outer social/environmental demands. Or to state it another way, to clarify the interactions of 'stress' (psychological) and 'press' (environmental) demands. In social work terms, person:environment interactions or person:environment fit.

A psychosocial assessment has a threefold FOCUS:

(1) The person, referring to the individual's personality system, particularly as it influences the individual's perception of and expectations for and reactions to situations; (2) the environment, including the concrete realities of the environment and its social psychological aspects; (3) person:environment interactions.

The OUTCOME of the assessment is an action plan designed to help strengthen the patient's capacity to cope with and to direct his or her own life.

The PURPOSES of such an assessment are: (1) to identify individual strengths and competencies which might be further developed to facilitate positively valued social interactions; (2) to identify areas of psychosocial stress and (3) to propose interventions that will lead to more satisfying person:environment fit given the patient's needs and level of functioning.

The GOALS of psychosocial assessment are to maximise the fit between person and environment so that the resident may live as close to normal life as possible and may participate in a way of life that supports his/her strengths and provides opportunities to build satisfying relationships.

The OBJECTIVE of the psychosocial assessment is to contribute information and knowledge of specific person:environment interactions to the treatment process and to address problems and issues surrounding a specific individual's social functioning.

Psychosocial stress refers to the mental and physiological reactions, produced by social conditions, that are detrimental to the long range adaptive functioning of an individual (Kaplan, Howard ed., 1983). Social conditions might include housing, nutrition, discrimination or oppression.

Mental reactions to stress can be ascertained by noting the presence of confusion in patients, their inability to perform tasks or focus on problems or a loss of memory. Clinically trained social workers learn to differentiate between normal, although extremely painful, adaptation to life-threatening situations, and the loss of adequate functioning; the difference between bereavement and pathological depression; recognise when someone slips from a depressive reaction into clinical depression.

Psychosocial assessments enhance their utility when complemented by the type of functional assessment outlined in Chapter 10 (Kuehn and McClain).

In keeping with a systems and generalist approach to social work practice, there are potentially four systems levels available for analysis. Changes in any one of these systems, or any combination of systems, could lead to the patient's enhanced social functioning and reduced psychosocial stress: the person:patient system; the family or substitute family system; the group or community system consisting of social networks and neighbourhood; and the institutional system constituted by laws, school, medical and social service agencies.

Four major areas noted to be sources of psychosocial stress, as well as sources of psychosocial well-being, are: (1) the presence or absence of social support, (2) the impact of *positive and negative life events or life changes* that either disrupt, or threaten to disrupt, an individual's usual activities; (3) the number and variety of roles and success in role performance (4) coping ability and style. Psychosocial assessment examines these four areas across the individual's spectrum of social interactions. This helps (a) identify areas where positive and validating transactions are taking place between person and environment, (b) identifies areas where support and modification of either person or environment are needed and (c) acts as a guide to help prevent interactions that may be inducing psychosocial stress.

It is this type of assessment in a hospital setting that furnishes the perspective which patients, families, medical staff, and interdisciplinary teams need in order to focus their vision on the way that people and environmental forces interact. The focus on these transactions, and ways to change them if necessary, has a direct impact on the quality of life a patient will experience during a hospital stay as well as during daily life long after the hospital stay is over.

Beyond the Clinical Social Work Role in Hospital Settings

Since social work began functioning in hospitals in the early 1900s, its stature and contributions to direct patient care have been increasingly recognised. As medicine moves away from a strictly disease model of practice and toward recognition of the importance interactions among biological, psychological and social factors play in an individual's health status, social work contributions become more visible and valued. As a result the roles social workers occupy in contemporary hospital social work practice have become more varied and demand a broader range of skills and knowledge.

For example, emphasis on shorter hospital stays and greater preference for care at home or in the community (in nursing and residential homes) have resulted in a greater stress on the function of discharge planning. Some practitioners maintain that planning for the appropriate and creative discharge of patients from hospital is the most critical and demanding clinical social work activity (Falck, 1989). The discharge planner's responsibility is to have a concrete discharge and follow-up plan in place prior to the patient's leaving the hospital. Social work involvement in discharge planning early in the hospital stay may reduce the length of stay in hospital, assure more-effective follow-up in the home or community, and enhance compliance with recommended regimens following discharge.

Since the 1970s when federal legislation required hospitals to establish ethics committees, social workers have been members of case consultation committees involved in the interdisciplinary process of ethical decision making. These committees also develop policies to address issues facing hospital staff in their treatment of certain populations, such as those having AIDS, patients in a persistent vegetative state, and patients wishing to terminate treatment (dialysis, respiratory, chemotherapy) or wishing to die by refusing food and water. The results of such committees have been of benefit to patients, families and the hospital as an institution. Social workers who initially served on these committees have not only enhanced their own sensitivity to ethical issues but they now are able to serve as consultants to community agencies, such as nursing homes, who wish to establish similar committees and procedures.

Another important role social workers in hospitals assume is that of training and educating patients, families, other hospital staff, and students from other disciplines who expect to become employed in health settings and the community at large. Education for the community is often provided through workshops, conferences and conventions for which registration fees are charged, thus generating revenues for the hospital.

Hospital social workers recognise that they cannot remain a valued participant in the field of health care unless they are contributing new information and knowledge, fresh insights and effective interventions designed to solve the problems facing patients and families and the health service delivery system. Social workers design projects and seek funding for a variety of research studies: descriptive and process studies; client satisfaction studies; effectiveness and/or outcome studies; programme evaluation studies; research on utilisation and accessibility of services; research into social epidemiology and screening instruments; research in quality and quantity assurance; and policy research (Berkman, 1983).

Conclusion
Modern medicine continues to move away from a strict disease orientation to the practice of medicine. There is increasing recognition of the role that the interaction of biological, psychological and social factors plays in an individual's or a population's health status. Working within this bio-psychosocial framework, social workers strongly grounded in their own profession's values, knowledge and skills and committed to their unique orientation to person:environment fit, will be increasingly valued for their contributions.

Notes
1. For a modern insight into interpersonal collaboration and conflict in corporate structure (and the hospital *is* a corporate structure) see Tribal Welfare in Organisations by Peg C. Neuhauser, Harper Collins, 1988.

References
Auberbach, Steven M.; Reported in Chicago Tribune, 8th September 1989.

Berkman, Barbara and Weissman, Andrew; 'Applied Social Research' ch. 6 in *Social Work and Health Care*; (eds) Miller, Rosalind and Rehr, Helen; 1983. NJ, Prentice Hall.

Carlton, Thomas Owen; *Clinical Social Work in Health Settings*; 1984: NY, Springer.

Cassell, Eric J.; 'The Nature of Suffering and the Goals of Medicine'. New England Journal of Medicine; Vol.306, 11 pp. 639 - 645; 1982.

Dana, Bess; 'The Collaborative Process' in (eds) Miller, Rosalind and Rehr: *Social Work Issues in Health Care*; 1983. NJ Prentice Hall.

Falck, Hans S.; 'Discharge Planning as Clinical Social Work'; Richmond: Virginia Commonwealth University, Richmond; 1989.

Germain, Carel B. and Gitterman, Alex; *The Life Model of Social Work Practice*. 1980. NY, Columbia University Press.

Golan, Naomi; *Treatment in Crisis Situations*; 1978. NY, Free Press.

Hartman, Ann and Laird, Joan; *Family Centred Social Work Practice*; 1983. NY, Free Press.

Jones, J.A. and Phillips, G.M.; *Communicating With Your Doctor.* 1988 Southern Illinois University Press: Carbondale.

Kaplan, Howard B.(ed.); *Psychosocial Stress*; 1983. NY, Academic Press.

Meyer, Carol; Social Work Practice. 1976. Free Press. London.

Meyer, Thos. and Abubaker, Walid; unpublished survey; St Mary's Hospital, Madison, Wisc., 1988.

Moos, Rudolph and Tsu,. V.O. (eds); *The Crisis of Physical Illness: an overview*; 1977. NY, Plenum Press.

Roberts, C. S.; 'Conflicting Professional Values in Social Work and Medicine'; in *Health Social Work*; 1989. Aug. 14 (3): p. 211-218.

Strauss, Anselm *et al.*; Chronic Illness and Quality of Life; 2nd ed., l984. St Louis, Mosby.

Tagliacozzo, Daisy L. and Mauksch, Hans O.; ' The Patient's View of the Patient's Role' in *Humanistic Health Care; Issues for Caregivers*; (eds.) Turner, G and Mapa, J; 1988. Ann Arbor, Mich.; Health Administration Press.

Turner, G and Mapa, J.; 'Part III: Practicing Humane Care – The Care Giver' in *Humanistic Health Care* (eds) Turner and Mapa; 1988. Ann Arbor, Mich. Health Administration Press.

Chapter 4
Oncology Social Work and Palliative Care in the United States

Matthew J. Loscalzo and James R. Zabora

The Evolution of Palliative Care

Cancer is universally experienced as an uncontrollable threat to existence and an assault on the integrity of the organism. Cancer generates conscious, unconscious and spiritual challenges inimical to the fulfilment of a meaningful present and future. Historically, no other illness has captured and maintained the fears and sense of dread as cancer. It is unique in its ability to simultaneously create a sense of uncontrollability and vulnerability. Cancer has come to symbolise the dark side of life and has supplanted previous symbols of dread and evil. Cancer bypasses conscious review and gains strength and momentum from myths, fears and fantasies. Yet cancer as the universal symbol of the inevitability of pain, suffering and death often unites people through the identification and acceptance of a common fate.

Kubler-Ross has provided a framework with which to understand the dying process (Kubler-Ross, 1969). This pioneering work created an environment in which the specific fears and underlying assumptions of the dying could be openly discussed. Kubler-Ross's work served to deepen the communication between those who confront death and those of us not yet in the front of the queue. In many ways her discussion of death mythology led to the humanisation of health care throughout the world.

The American psyche has as its foundation the western European belief that men and women can overcome all obstacles and that the natural world can be exploited and controlled if adequate resources are available. Cancer is seen as but one more uncontrollable natural force to be overcome. In many ways cancer is perceived as the confrontation of this belief, the Vietnam of medical science. The American response to cancer has been as vociferous as it has been frustrating. The 'war on cancer' has claimed many victims and led to mistrust of the 'system' in spite of some significant victories.

Twenty years into this 'war' the perception is that there is no end in sight, even though recent major advances in molecular biology hold the promise of a genetic cure and vaccine. The potential for universal genetic screening has also dramatically increased. This genetic screening, which will be able to predict many illnesses prior to birth, presents enormous and complex ethical challenges to social workers dedicated to assuring that consumers of services receive the benefits, rather than become the victims, of these futuristic innovations.

There has recently been a re-emphasis on the unity of the mind and body of patients with cancer. These changes are a direct result of (1) the consumer movements of the 1970s and 1980s, in which patients and families demanded to play an increasingly active role in health care delivery and policy; (2) their demands for compassionate or humanistic 'science with a heart'; (3) the impact of modern cognitive psychological research which links cognitions to mood and to immune functioning; (4) extensive governmental, corporate and public concern over the rising costs of medical care in a rapidly ageing population.

There is enhanced appreciation for the psychological and social milieu of the patient and family but cost considerations almost always supersede the medical and psychosocial needs of the general population. This presents a quandary for the American people: is health care a right or privilege? how should individual needs be evaluated viz-à-viz societal costs? and above all – who will pay?

Within this overall context of American health care lies the care and treatment of those affected by cancer. Cancer statistics for the United States, published in 1988, are sobering: 50 per cent mortality within five years; 500,000 deaths each year. The struggles of cancer patients, their families and those who provide care, symbolise the very best of what it means to be 'human'.

Oncology social workers participate in the care and study of people with tumours. Their primary concern is for those affected by cancer. They are involved in the process of clinical care, advocacy, education and applied research. Specifically, social workers attend to the psychological, practical, social, educational and informational needs of patients and their families through (1) counselling, (2) information gathering and interpretation, (3) resource engagement, (4) advocacy, (5) programme development and (6) community organisation.

Hospice Care and Its Relationship to Palliative Care
  Palliative care is the active total care of patients whose disease is not responsive to curative treatment. Control of pain, of other symptoms and of psychological, social and spiritual problems is paramount. The goal of palliative care is achievement of the best possible quality of life for patients and their families. Palliative care had its origins in the hospice movement (European Journal of Palliative Care, 1989).

Oncology Social Work and Palliative Care in the United States

In 1982 the United States Congress passed an amendment to the Social Security Act providing for payment of hospice care for those over age 65 and those permanently disabled. Although the hospice movement was well established in Great Britain (Sanders, 1978), this legislation recognised the unique needs of terminally ill patients in the United States for the first time. Since the hospice movement emanated from grass roots (especially well-organised elderly people) this programme was separate and distinct from that of organised medicine. Free-standing community-based programmes were quickly established. They offered solace, pain management, and family support. However, unlike their European counterparts these programmes cared for dying patients predominantly in the patient's own home.

The quality of care initially provided by these free-standing community-based hospices was inconsistent. While some hospices provided state of the art care, others were under-funded, had undertrained staff and provided for little more than the most basic comfort needs. Today there are over 2,100 organisations providing hospice services in the United States, a National Hospice Organization exists and national standards have been created.

The early focus of services and this model of hospice care were self-limiting. By the mid-1970s it was apparent that this model of care needed to be expanded and integrated into that of general medical practice (Ventafridda). This led to loose alliances between community-based hospices and local community hospitals and an expanded definition of terminal illness which included those who had a prognosis of six months or less.

Out of experience with this group of patients emerged the palliative care model, a model of service which was to subsume hospice as but one significant aspect of care. Emphasis on palliative care provided the means to again reunite the needs of the chronically ill with the benefits of established medical institutions. This comprehensive type of palliative care is the speciality providing focused medical, nursing, psychological, social and spiritual care.

Relieved of the burden of cure, care focuses on (1) maximising quality of life, (2) effective symptom management and (3) comprehensive rehabilitation within the context of chronic illness and disability at all stages of the illness. Within the context of the American mythology around the omnipotence of conquering disease through science, palliative care represents a distinct ongoing evolution in *how* medical service and *what* medical services are valued and provided. This shift in focus and spending, from *curing* to *caring*, could occur only in the context of a rapidly ageing and well-organised populace whose voices are heard through consumer involvement. Patients and families now require and demand the very best of medical science and 'state of the art' symptom management and rehabilitation at all stages of the illness process.

The social work roles of mental health counsellor, educator and advocate are essential to this comprehensive model of care.

The Social Work Role in Clinical Care

Although there are a few significant exceptions[1], virtually all oncology social workers function in a health care setting, not a social service setting. Within this framework psychological, social and practical services are provided as part of overall medical care and costs for these services are calculated as part of the overall cost of medical care.

Social work services are generally provided in order to optimise the patient's response to treatment. When practical needs expand much beyond the context of their medical care, patients are referred to appropriate resources. The foci of individual oncology social workers vary but have these basic elements: (1) clinical care or service, (2) education and (3) research. This emphasis mirrors the settings in which the majority of oncology social workers function and the cultural milieu of those settings.

Since the early nineteenth century the importance of psychosocial variables — especially those of housing, sanitation, employment and family health — and their relationship to medical outcomes has been increasingly recognised. The importance of the social milieu to which the patients return after medical treatment is also seen as a significant influence on continued medical improvement. Oncology social workers focus on maximising the quality of life of each patient, no matter whether newly diagnosed or terminally ill, and serve as the bridge for learning how to maintain as normal a life as possible.

Quality of Life: Clinical Care

The primary clinical foci of oncology social workers include: (1) psychological screening, (2) assessment, (3) counselling, (4) referral when needed, and (5) attending to practical needs. Services are provided through individual, family and group modalities. Interventions tend to be short term, practical and problem centred. Table I details social work interventions within a continuity of care model.

Table I Oncology Social Work

Psychosocial Screening Phase	• Co-ordinates screening to identify high distress patients. • Receives referrals for high distress patients and families in need of psychotherapy.
Diagnostic Phase	• Provides crisis intervention or short-term therapy to moderate to high distress patients. • Provides linkage to community resources • Provides long-term counselling or psychotherapy to patients and families with severe psychosocial histories.
Treatment Phase	• Provides short-term therapy, relaxation techniques and support to facilitate adaptation to the diagnosis and treatment. • Teaches specific coping skills to relieve anxiety and physical discomfort. • Assists with referrals to community resources for specific needs. • Provides discharge planning for patients with complex needs. • Provides ongoing long-term psychotherapy to patients and families. • Addresses severe psychosocial problems such as substance abuse and sexual abuse.
Follow-up	• Provides short-term therapy or crisis intervention as needed. • Develops, co-ordinates and facilitates patient and family support groups with appropriate team members. • Acts as liaison between patient and resources as needed. • Provides additional information concerning cancer support programmes and other community resources. • Tends to the practical, psychological and social needs of the dying and family. • Provides support to bereaved families • Continues long-term psychotherapy or counselling to resolve significant problem areas • Counsels families re: long-term issues exacerbated by the patient's cancer diagnosis

In the United States approximately 84 per cent of the supportive counselling provided to cancer patients and their families is provided by social workers (Ventafridda, 1988). Significantly, but not surprisingly, the three primary concerns and fears of patients and families in order of importance to them are: (1) disruption to family life, (2) death, and (3) uncontrollable pain (Coluzzi, submitted). However, lack of control over an uncertain future and fear of abandonment are often the most significant underlying yet unspoken fears of cancer patients and their families. Financial concerns are often of grave concern to patients and families alike, as income is often drastically reduced during chronic medical illness. Money is often seen as an instrument of power and may be experienced as a metaphor for control (Levin *et al.*, 1985). In addition, the overwhelming demands of the illness and of the complex medical bureaucratic system itself may synergistically join to thwart efforts to maintain a patient's and family's sense of control over what is happening in their lives.

Psychosocial treatments have been shown to reduce depression, anxiety and stress; to be cost effective; to improve coping skills; and improve quality of life for the medically ill (Farkas, 1987). Anxiety, depression, agitation, helplessness, powerlessness and hopelessness are common reactions to cancer and its noxious treatments. Significant clinical depression is prevalent in 6 per cent of patients in primary care treatment settings and in 11 per cent of medical in-patients (Katon, Sullivan, 1990). Forty-seven per cent of patients with cancer fit the criteria for a psychiatric diagnosis. However, even within the majority of cancer patients free from a psychiatric diagnosis, expectable psychological reactions of intense fear, isolation and financial distress are a direct result of a life-threatening illness (Derogatis *et al.*, 1983).

Physically, common effects resulting from disfiguring surgeries and toxic chemotherapeutic agents may lead to permanent impaired cognitive and physical functioning. Cancer invades the bone, muscle and nerve which may result in intractable pain, permanent disability, and death.

Clearly, all cancer patients require some type of psychosocial intervention or support. It is the social worker's role to work with the patient and family to jointly delineate any barriers to insuring that the patient fully benefits from medical treatment. Secondarily, it is the social worker's responsibility to offer the opportunity to the patient and family to attend to any other psychological, social or practical problems which manifest themselves as a barrier to their optimal functioning. Common examples of these barriers include: untreated mental illness, substance abuse, unsafe housing, unemployment and overwhelming family conflict. Table II outlines some of the common reactions resulting from the cancer experience.

Table II. Common Reactions to the Cancer Experience

Medical Event	Possible Reactions
Initial diagnosis	Crisis reaction
Diagnosis workups	Anxiety reactions to medical testing Acute pain Stress reaction
Medical interventions (surgery, chemotherapy,	Acute pain related to treatments Anxiety reactions related to pain, discomfort, prognosis radiation therapy) Stress reactions Anticipatory nausea and vomiting Avoidance of treatment Depression
Remission	Anxiety, hypochondriasis Depression Family strain
Terminal illness	Chronic pain Anxiety reactions Depression Suffering Family strain Agitation
Bereavement	Anxiety reactions Insomnia Guilt reactions Depression

Quality of Life: Family Relationships
Since social support is a critical variable in the patient's adaptation, the family most often and effectively fulfils this essential role. This is especially true of the patient with advanced disease. Managing a long, protracted illness followed by imminent death strikes at the very fabric of the family system. Psychological, social, spiritual and financial support systems are at significant risk for breakdown. The changes are multilevel and always complex. Attempts have been made to quantify social support by an objective examination of pertinent

variables such as marital status, living arrangements, availability of family members and other relatives (Weisman et al., 1980). Table III outlines social support and other variables associated with psychosocial adaptation.

Table III. Variables Associated with Psychosocial Adaptation (19)

SOCIAL SUPPORT	PAST HISTORY	CURRENT CONCERNS
Marital Status	Substance Abuse	Health
Education	Depression	Living Arrangements
Living Arrangements	Mental Health	Work
Employment	Major Illnesses	Finances
Relatives Nearby	Physical Symptoms	Friends
Neighbours	Cancer's Course	Existential Concerns
Church Attendance	Past Regrets	Self-Appraisal
	Optimism v Pessimism	

However, a quantitative description does not equate with the ability of any family system to actually provide the support which a patient needs. In some instances, families may attempt to provide too much support and this may disrupt a patient's attempt to successfully adapt to their illness (Berkman et al., 1992). For example, family members may attempt to protect the patient by encouraging them to delay participation in painful physical therapy to prevent muscular atrophy or encourage too early a return to eating after dietary restrictions. In addition, the patient with advanced disease and uncontrolled symptoms such as pain and delirium, can create a sense of chaos which may threaten the integrity of the family structure. It is within the purview of social work to identify and evaluate the quality of support provided by the family. This is often most effectively achieved through a home visit to assess patient and family functioning in their natural setting.

Family literature provides a range of theories to describe how functioning occurs within families. Family unity (Geismar, 1964), enmeshment (Minuchin, 1974), and cross-generational alliances (Haley, 1963) are concepts which describe certain aspects of family behaviour. The Circumplex Model of Family Functioning (Olson, 1988) focuses on two of the most salient family constructs, that is, adaptability and cohesion. This model can be helpful in the medical setting to assess the resources and limitations of the family system. Methods exist which actually measure these critical variables and possess highly acceptable levels of reliability and validity. If possible, psychosocial screening should also be undertaken to prospectively identify families which might present difficulties for the health care team to manage. Brief pencil and paper tests identifying patients and families who are the most in need for social work intervention can insure the most efficient use of these services.

Social workers are usually perceived by the health care team as the identified person to work with families. This unique opportunity enables the social worker to gain an in-depth understanding of the patient and family milieu and to develop treatment plans tailored to their individual needs.

Adaptability and Cohesion
Adaptability can be defined as the capability of any family to reorganise or restructure itself when confronted by a stressful event. Under significant stress, families need to reassign internal roles, modify rules for daily living and/or revise their decision-making process. While many families accept this challenge, approximately 30 per cent of all families cannot adapt and consequently may be a loss or a disruption to the health care team (Zabora, 1989).

On the other hand, *cohesion* is the amount of emotional bonding which exists between family members. Cohesion can be high, moderate or low. High cohesion tends to suggest enmeshment in families where little autonomy exists for each individual member. Low cohesion or minimal emotional bonding expresses a lack of commitment to other family members. These families may be unavailable to medical staff for support of the patient or as participants in the decision-making process (Zabora, 1992).

Often in the care of the patient and family, early indicators suggest which families may be an asset or a liability to caring for a patient. Early indicators of family adjustment include: seeking information appropriately, providing support to the patient, visiting regularly, assisting with activities of daily living, facilitating medical treatment plans, possessing a positive attitude, demonstrating support to one another, focusing on patient rather than family needs.

Early identification which is combined with a comprehensive family assessment maximises the health care team's ability to respond to a wide range of the behaviour exhibited by diverse family types. Interactions between the team and family members during the diagnostic and initial treatment phases set the stage for ongoing contact. Specific interventions of the team include: (1) information giving, (2) emotional support, (3) availability and (4) the instilling of a sense of hope and concern. Such interventions provide the opportunity to build an effective alliance with the family on behalf of the patient.

Family Life Cycle

A final consideration within Olson's Circumplex Model is the concept of the Family Life Cycle. Critical to the family life cycle concept is its dynamic nature. Daily living within families generates normal stressors. As a result, overall marital satisfaction, family satisfaction and quality of life are also in a constant state of flux. Normal changes or stressors may intensify if the family cannot respond to tasks at each developmental stage. *Adaptability* and *cohesion* levels play critical roles in relation to how successfully families move through the life cycle. Within this framework unanticipated stressful events, such as a cancer diagnosis, can occur and disrupt a family's natural transition from one stage to the next.

The diagnosis of cancer within a family severely disrupts the normal course of events in a family's life cycle. Olson has labelled seven stages in the family life cycle: (1) young couples without children; (2) families with pre-schoolers; (3) families with school age children; (4) families with adolescents (age thirteen to eighteen); (5) families with children age nineteen or older who are launching their own families; (6) families whose children have left home; (7) families in retirement. A range of variables determine the family's response. For example, the response of a family at Stage 1 (young couples with no children) may be quite different from a family at Stage 5 (children leaving home).

In summary, factors such as a family's level of adaptability and cohesion in conjunction with the stage in the life cycle greatly influence a family's response to a prolonged life-threatening disease. Families may be temporarily impaired, or if their functioning is already in an extreme category, their behaviour may be problematic to the health care team.

Quality of Life: Coping with Pain and Suffering

Cancer patients frequently manifest a variety of physical and psychological symptoms as direct effects of cancer and its treatments. Social workers aid in the management of these symptoms. Commonly identified symptoms include: acute and chronic pain, anxiety, insomnia, hypochondriasis, anticipatory nausea and vomiting, and depression. Anorexia and asthenia are also major concerns. Although not exhaustive, Table II lists some of the most common and expected psychosocial reactions which confront cancer patients and their families.

To varying degrees cognitive behavioural and other psychosocial approaches can ameliorate these unpleasant symptoms. Unfortunately, symptoms such as anorexia or asthenia are a major concern. They negatively affect large numbers of patients in ways which are inimical to their overall health and compliance with medical care. Despite the anxiety of patients, and especially in families where food may have been a highly invested mode of communication, symptoms such as anorexia are understudied, are rarely identified as significant problems, and are seldom referred for psychological, nutritional or medical treatment.

Cancer-related pain, nausea and vomiting and anxiety represent some of the most common noxious symptoms experienced by cancer patients. Affective, behavioural, motivational and perceptual variables significantly influence these symptoms. Consequently, cognitive-behavioural techniques emerge as the focal approach for the treatment of these symptoms.

Social workers are in a unique position to teach cognitive-behavioural interventions to patients and families thereby enabling them to have a repertoire of coping skills available when needed. These coping skills are helpful in managing emotional reactions and tolerating medical tests and treatments.

Although psychosocial variables such as anxiety, depression, fear, and feelings of powerlessness and hopelessness may exacerbate a patient's cancer pain experience, the relationship is not causal (Foley, 1985). Therefore the teaching of coping skills by the social worker can support hope and mastery in the face of uncontrollable factors secondary to the illness and its treatment. During the diagnostic and treatment phases patients and families require ongoing information and support. After active treatment, the patient often needs to learn specific coping skills.

Basic Principles of Cognitive-Behavioural Interventions
Cognitive-behavioural approaches originate with the laws of learning and conditioning. They are based on the same principles, expanded to include mentation, explored so extensively by Nobel Laureate Pavlov at the turn of the century. Through an adequate appreciation for the importance of the interaction between the patient's thoughts, feeling and behaviours and the interaction of these with the social environment, a variety of cognitive and behavioural interventions can be systematically employed to enhance an individual's coping ability (Turk, *et al.*, 1983). Patients' activities, whether they are thoughts, feelings or behaviour, can be socially rewarded or encouraged. As a result physical tension, distress or pain can be reduced.

Usually interactions between patients and their families produce the vast majority of reinforcing, inhibiting or extinguishing responses. Consequently, a cognitive-behavioural treatment plan actively engages and integrates key family members into the implementation of strategies to resolve the problematic symptom. Exclusion of the patient's primary care giver in treatment planning often results in family resistance. Loss of the family as ally in treatment is even more significant if the patient is significantly impaired, possesses advanced disease, or is terminally ill. For the health care provider, it should be emphasised that cognitive-behavioural approaches enable cancer patients and their families to maximise their sense of control and hope — feelings which are often the first and second casualties following a cancer diagnosis. This is especially true for patients requiring palliative care.

Since cancer patients and families pass through different phases following their diagnosis, this necessitates revisions of goals and treatment plans so that the specific needs of each patient can be met at each phase. Over the course of the illness, the most common needs are: (1) maintenance of quality of life, (2) attention to mood, (3) acquisition of coping skills and (4) reduction in suffering (Bandura, 1977).

Cancer Pain as a Model for Effective Intervention
Cancer pain is present in nearly 75 per cent of cancer patients with advanced disease and 90 per cent of patients with terminal cancer (Daut, l982). Cancer-related pain and its associated distress provide an acceptable paradigm in which to apply cognitive-behavioural approaches for general use with all cancer patients and their families. There is considerable literature on medical aspects of managing cancer pain (Foley, 1985). Psychological approaches to cancer pain are relatively new treatments which have become available to patients and families to supplement medical management of cancer pain (Turk, 1992).

Commonly used cognitive-behavioural interventions include: (1) relaxation techniques (breathing and muscular); (2) distraction; (3) hypnosis and visual imagery; (4) correcting cognitive distortions; (5) desensitisation; (6) graded task assignments; (7) assertiveness training; and (8) differential reinforcement. These interventions teach skills to both patients and families, who have an opportunity to practise them until a sense of mastery is attained. Inexpensive audiotape recorders are often utilised to encourage practice and enhance compliance.

As an adjunct to medical care, cognitive-behavioural interventions promote optimal functioning and rehabilitation through the encouragement of active participation of patients and family members in the control of symptoms and the acquisition of specific skills which increase hope and expand the the patient's and family's belief in their ability to accomplish the tasks needed to reach therapeutic goals. These interventions, however, are never a substitute for appropriate and comprehensive medical management (Cleeland, 1984).

Guidelines for Referrals

Following the diagnostic phase, exploration of necessity for referral to other agencies and services, psychosocial assessment and other salient issues, the potential uses of cognitive-behavioural approaches should be explored and, if appropriate, intervention should begin as soon as possible.

Since palliative care patients tend to experience pain and other debilitating symptoms more often than other patients, the role of the social worker as advocate and teacher of skills is especially significant. In essence, social workers can employ cognitive-behavioural skills to empower patients and families and to minimise suffering and hopelessness.

Quality of Life: Sexuality

Social workers often have the opportunity to foster open communication concerning this significant barrier to quality of life. It is the social worker's role to create an environment where this discussion can occur.

Advances in cancer treatments continue to increase and extend survival. As a result cancer patients need help in normalising their daily lives. This normalising helps to achieve optimal physical, psychological, and social functioning (Mantell, 1982). Sexuality and intimacy are important in varying degrees to all people regardless of age and diagnosis. Generally, the biggest barrier to the open discussion of changes in sexual function and intimacy resides within the health care community. Sexual functioning is a critical concept in the physical, psychological, and social rehabilitation of cancer patients given that all cancers possess the capability to affect body image and/or self-esteem. Therefore, decrease in sexual functioning and perceptions of sexual attractiveness can diminish patients' overall sense of well-being (Wise, 1980).

Timely recognition of patients' sexual needs and dysfunctions is essential to comprehensive cancer care. Given the nature of advanced disease and its treatment the social worker can make a major contribution to patient and family control and comfort by attending to these concerns. Unfortunately, health professionals often stress survival and control of the disease and ignore sexuality as an essential aspect related to the quality of life of the cancer patient.

Patients may also be reluctant to raise sexual issues as a concern because they are embarrassed to discuss this intimate topic. Fears that cancer is contagious through sexual activity, that having sex may cause a recurrence, that cancer is a punishment for past sexual misconduct, or that a sexual partner may be exposed to radiation if the patient is receiving external beam radiation therapy are but a few of the commonly held misunderstandings (Wasow, 1982). The emergence of AIDS as an epidemic has made discussion of sexuality and intimacy even more difficult.

To address these misconceptions and to engage in a total psychosocial rehabilitation of the cancer patient, health care personnel need to conduct a sexual assessment as part of their routine care. A health review of the vital systems of the body with routine questions about eating, smoking, drinking, and sleeping habits ought to include specific inquiries about sexual functioning and relationships. Asking questions about sexuality within this context normalises these concerns and creates an environment where they can be openly discussed. Often the patient and family look to the social worker for permission and guidance to discuss these concerns.

A comprehensive clinical assessment must take an orderly approach to systematically ascertain the role of sexuality for each cancer patient. A large proportion of sexual dysfunctions have psychological as well as physiological origins so it is important to differentiate between the anatomic changes and the emotional effects of the disease. Even when sexual functioning is disrupted by physiological processes, psychological support and guidance are important. Possible *psychological effects include*: regression due to the sick role; lowered self-esteem; fears of appearance — scars, odours, amputations; comfort minimised by pain; and agility and/or mobility limited by disease or treatment (Wise, 1980).

Organic limitations, on the other hand, are easily divided into two categories: (1) endogenous, which are attributed to the disease effects, and (2) exogenous, which are drug or treatment induced.

Quality of Life: Spirituality[2] and Survivorship
One salient aspect associated with the distress of life-threatening or terminal illness is one's spiritual self-awareness. Studies concerned with spiritual well-being (Reed, 1987), spiritual coping strategies (Sodestrom, 1987), and the relationship of spiritual well-being to hope (Carson *et al.*, 1988) indicate that an awareness of spirituality should be fundamental to the study of psychosocial distress related to any life-threatening or terminal illness. Many traditional western psychologies, however, fail to recognise spirituality and transcendental needs as intrinsic aspects of human nature (Bodian, 1989). Therefore, providers of psychosocial services may not meet the needs of those facing a life-threatening or terminal illness.

An essential principle for meaningful intervention with these populations is the fundamental perspective that as human beings we are far more than either the sum of our biological parts or the influence of our environment. Acknowledgement of the spiritual aspect of the person is based on the principle that there are powerful forces within the psyche which propel us toward greater wholeness and integration. Bodian describes this journey as a potential psychospiritual transformation beyond the ego. However, traditional theories of psychology underlying many psychosocial interventions are highly dependent on ego psychology and as a result lack a theoretical framework for an ego-transcending phenomenon such as death. Therefore, those facing a life-threatening illness often approach dying and death from a fearful and reactive stance. However, people can be helped to accept their own mortality within a framework which normalises death.

Whether or not a prognosis of death is ever indicated, clinicians observe that cancer patients, at the time of diagnosis and throughout their illness, enter a process of exploring what life and death mean to them. As they begin this exploration, traditional values and spiritual belief systems are questioned and challenged. A redefinition of one's attitude towards death may be necessary in order to formulate a personal death perspective that serves as a comfort rather than a threat. If the patient is able to move beyond commonly held beliefs, this developmental task can be accomplished. However, this interactive process of formulating a personal death perspective and a heightened spiritual awareness can generate elevated levels of distress to cancer patients and their families. If a patient is unable to find a comforting death perspective, or if the level of spiritual orientation is inadequate, the patient may experience significant psychosocial distress. Higher levels of spirituality are associated with an increase in a patient's ability to normalise death and patients who accomplish this task experience lower levels of psychosocial distress (Smith *et al.*, 1993)..

As with sexuality, spirituality is an essential life-affirming force which is often ignored or denied within a medical context. The social worker may help identify the characteristics of spiritual life and use them to help patients explore a spiritual perspective which will help maintain a sense of well-being in the face of a life-threatening illness and death. For those with religious faith, clergy may become an important part of the health-care team.

Survivorship
Due to recent technological advances in the detection and treatment of cancer, nearly half of the people diagnosed with these life-threatening diseases are expected to be alive five years later. Increasing numbers of cancer patients are now either cured of their disease or live for many years with their disease, but they face

the complex process of adjusting to life after cancer treatment. This has created a growing population of cancer survivors who have successfully completed their cancer treatment but live with a number of specialised needs.

A number of studies indicate that while survival may be achieved, cancer is still a disease that can substantially affect several physical and psychological aspects of a survivor's life. These physical and psychological 'late effects' appear to result from (1) the physical complications of aggressive cancer treatments, (2) the stress of being near death, and (3) the stigmatising effects of being labelled a cancer patient (Ganz, *et al.*, 1986).

Survivors have to deal with problems related to being in a dependent patient role and this generates difficulty in returning to pre-illness roles. Cancer survivors and their family members seldom escape the ongoing fear of recurrence. Hypervigilance and hypochondriasis are common reactions which should be addressed at every opportunity.

Cancer survivors generally experience challenges in four critical life domains: (1) physical health: (2) psychological and social well-being: (3) maintaining adequate health insurance: and (4) employment. Physical health challenges for cancer survivors include a fear of recurrence, the possibility of a secondary malignancy and other late medical effects of aggressive treatments. Many survivors actively strive to meet these challenges by maintaining their physical health through preventive regimens of diet, exercise, stress reduction and smoking cessation. These activities restore some sense of control to the cancer survivor in the realm of their physical health.

Psychological and social well-being of cancer survivors is challenged in other ways. While no two cancer survivors respond in the exact same way, emotions frequently confronted include: elation to be finishing treatment, residual shock, anger, grief, sadness and existential questioning. In general, most cancer survivors report mild to moderate levels of psychological distress. Those patients who lack social support, have a previous psychiatric history, have severe physical limitations or who have a pattern of maladaptive coping may experience even higher levels of distress and will be impeded in their adjustment to survivorship.

The maintenance of adequate health insurance coverage is extremely important to cancer survivors. However, cancer survivors are often threatened with policy cancellations or reductions in coverage. Furthermore, the linkage of job and insurance creates difficulties for survivors who feel compelled to retain their current employment rather than risk the possibility of losing their health care coverage.

Finally, employment issues which concern cancer survivors centre around failure to be promoted, negative attitudes toward cancer and undue criticism from supervisors or co-workers. Few cancer patients actually encounter dismissal from their place of employment, but a larger number experience the more subtle difficulties as described above.

Because the bulk of the survivorship literature tends to cluster around the four domains of challenge set forth above, a number of programmes are being established to address the specialised needs of this population. The National Cancer Institute has developed a booklet as a guide for cancer survivors entitled Facing Forward which addresses these four domains (National Cancer Institute, 1990).

The Social Work Role in Patient and Family Education
Due to the nature and treatment of a chronic life-threatening illness, patients and families consistently require information concerning all aspects of their care. As hospitals increasingly serve patients in out-patient settings and home care is expanded, the need to enhance patient and family education will increase. Social workers use and assess educational material and may help develop new materials when needed, often as part of an interdisciplinary team.

Numerous studies have demonstrated that educational materials and consent forms are poorly written, confusing and at a reading level well above what patients and families can comprehend. Educational materials must be developed to address the specific informational requirements of the patient and family. Materials should reflect consideration of the specific disease, its site, stage, state of progression, and treatment modalities. They must be designed to the level of comprehension and education of ordinary people. At minimum, audio cassette tapes, television, videotapes, talking books, passive and interactive computer assisted learning must all be tailored to the population at large. Engagement of patients and families in the development of particular learning material, especially in language other than English, may insure acceptability by the population to be served. Group work with patients and family members in the hospital and community provides an effective arena for the use and development of some educational materials, such as videos or other films.

The Social Work Role in Research
Clinical effectiveness can only be enhanced through the evaluation of social work practice. In order to evaluate their practice, social workers must understand and learn to comfortably use standard research methods.

For many years recommendations for systematic evaluation of social work outcomes have been ignored. If clinical interventions seek to reduce anxiety or depression, or to improve family relationships, or enhance quality of life, the extent to which these outcomes are achieved must be reliably measured by valid criteria (Coulton, 1979). Without incorporation of research methods into clinical practice, demonstrations that a specific outcome (such as a decrease in anxiety) is a product of a social work intervention are extremely difficult.

Research also contributes to the social work knowledge base. In many respects the social work profession has borrowed theoretical perspectives from the fields of sociology, psychology and economics to guide its practice. In order to fully sustain identification and acceptance as a profession, the social work field must move towards the creation and maintenance of its own knowledge base and enhance its ability to be accountable.

Finally, research serves a valuable purpose in relation to overall job satisfaction. Social workers who provide services to the chronically and terminally ill can experience depression, guilt, helplessness, insecurity and grief as a direct result of clinical relationships with their patients and families (Vachon, 1987).

Research provides an opportunity for a problem to be studied and, as a result, clinical practices may be revised. In some cases, projects may result in the publication of abstracts or manuscripts. These activities not only produce long-term gratification, they provide some assurance that interventions undertaken in daily practice are contributing to the overall understanding of the presenting problem and may make life better for those in the future.

Social workers possess the insight needed to contribute to important research designed to better understand concepts such as psychosocial screening, the impact of illness on the family, the effectiveness of relaxation techniques and measurement of quality of life issues.

Conclusion
Importance of Oncology Social Work
In the evolution of medicine there was an initial need to split the whole person into mind and body in order to more accurately study physical attributes. This separation of the body from the mind depersonalises illness and allows health care providers to focus only on the physical elements of disease. Partialisation of the body into its many systems and subsystems enables biofunctioning to be studied in its most minute detail. Unfortunately, during this process the individual personality attached to the body is often ignored and thought to be of little consequence to treatment outcomes.

In recent years, there has been a strong movement to revisit reductionistic methods of science and medicine and to heal the dichotomy of the mind:body split. There has been a call to view the patient in totality, to restore the personality to the body, and to once again consider the total human being. In doing so, the physical aspects of illness become only one part of a larger system that needs to be targeted for intervention. The psychological impact of illness now comes into question as well as the social consequences. Spirituality as a fundamental attribute of the human condition adds a further dimension for assessment and intervention. All four quadrants of the person — the physical, the mental, the emotional and the spiritual — with their attendant social influences, come into play in defining the illness experience. These influences, typically known as psychosocial factors, have become extremely important in understanding the physiological processes of disease and illness.

Multidisciplinary Approach

In providing comprehensive care that addresses all aspects of illness a multidisciplinary team approach is essential. With the partialisation of medicine into specialities and sub-specialities, any comprehensive model of care requires a team approach. In this approach, a number of professionals with their unique expertise must come together to provide the necessary care for each quadrant of the individual (physical, mental, emotional or spiritual) with respect to the particular cancer diagnosis and stage of illness. Certainly medicine is moving in the direction of distinguishing between 'disease' as a physical process and 'illness' as more inclusive of the influence of other human attributes. Therefore health care providers who seek to treat illness must incorporate psychosocial rehabilitation into routine care.

This comprehensive and unified approach to illness is quickly becoming the model of care in oncology. The role of the social worker within this model is to provide (1) psychological counselling, (2) advocacy and (3) assistance with practical barriers to medical care.

Technology Transfer

There is a great deal of knowledge related to the field of psychosocial oncology. The gaps in our ability to truly understand the full impact of cancer on patients and families are equally impressive. However, one must ask to what extent our knowledge has been operationalised into specific clinical interventions or services. Certainly, there are excellent examples such as cognitive-behavioural interventions and the development of psychoeducational sessions for cancer survivors. How much of our knowledge has actually been transferred into practice? To what extent is it applied? Are health care providers obligated to employ these techniques? Such questions are critical to the field of social work.

As some countries move toward a new century of futuristic cancer treatments such as gene therapy, others are desperately struggling to provide basic supportive care for curable diseases. However, for oncology social workers the essential question is the same. How do we humanise medical care in the face of many complex countervailing forces? Social workers must work with other professionals to ensure that patients and families are not lost in the struggle. The search for the humanising integration of body, mind, spirit and family must continue everywhere.

Notes

1. Cancer Care Incorporated, located in New York City, is a free-standing social work agency providing social work services to patients and families.

2. 'Spiritual' refers to those aspects of human life relating to expeiences that transcend sensory phenomena. It may have a religious base for some but for many others spirituality is associated mainly with meaning and purpose, forgiveness, reconciliation and affirmation of worth.

References

Bandura, A.: Self-efficacy: Toward a Unifying Theory of Behavioural Change; *Psych. Rev.* 84:191, 1977.

Berkman L., Leo-Summers I., Horwitz R.I.: Emotional Support and Survival After Myocardial Infarction. *Annals of Internal Medicine* 117(12):1003, 1992.

Bodian S.: If Buddha Had Been a Shrink; *Yoga Journal*, Sept. Oct. 1989.

Carson V., Soeken K., Grimm P.: Hope and Its Relationship to Spiritual Well Being. *Journal of Psychology and Theology* 6(2): 159, 1988.

Cleeland C.S.: The Impact of Pain on the Patient with Cancer. Cancer, 54:2635, 1984.

Coluzzi P.H., Grant M., Doroshow J.H., Rhiner M., Ferrell B. and Rivera L. *Survey of the Provision of Supportive Care Services at National Cancer Institute. Designated Cancer Centers*, Submitted for publication.

Coulton, Claudia J.: *Social Work Quality Assurance Programs: A Comparative Analysis*; Silver Spring, NASW, Inc., 1979.

Daut R.L., Cleeland C.S.: The Prevalence and Severity of Pain in Cancer. *Cancer* 50(9)1913, 1982.

Derogatis L.R., Morrow G.R., Fetting J. et al., The Prevalence of Psychiatric Disorders Among Cancer Patients. *JAMA* 1983; 249; 751-757.

European Journal of Palliative Care, Newsletter 1; 1989.

Farkas C., Loscalzo M.: Death Without Indignity. In A. H. Kutscher, A. C. Carr and L.G. Kutscher, eds *Principles of Thanatology*. New: Columbus University Press, 1987.

Foley, K.M.: The Treatment of Cancer Pain. N. Engl. *Journal. Med.* 13:84, 1985.

Ganz P.A., Rofessard J., Polinsky M.L., et al.: A Comprehensive Approach to Cancer Patients' Needs Assessment: The Cancer Inventory of Problem Situations (CIPS) and a Companion Interview. *Journal of Psychosocial Oncology* 4(3):75, 1986.

Geismar L.L., La Sorte M.A.: *Understanding the Multi-Problem Family*. New York: Associated Press, l964.

Haley J.: *Strategies of Psychotherapy*. New York: Grune and Stratton, 1963.

Katon W., Sullivan M.D., Depression and Chronic Medical Illness. *Journal of Clinical Psychiatry* 1990; 56(suppl.): 3 - 11.

Kubler-Ross E., *On Death and Dying*. New York: MacMillan, 1969.

Levin D.N., Cleeland C.S., Dar R.: Public attitudes toward cancer pain. *Cancer* 56:2337, 1985.

Mantell J.E., *Sexuality and Cancer: Psychosocial Aspects of Cancer*. New York: Raven Press, 1982.

Minuchin S.: *Families and Family Therapy*. Cambridge, Mass: Harvard University Press, 1974.

National Cancer Institutue: *Facing Forward: A Guide for Cancer Survivors.*Washington, D.C.: US. Dept of Health and Human Services, National Institute of Health, July, 1990.

Olson D.H., Sprenkle R.H. (eds): *Circumplex Model: Systemic Assessment and Treatment of Families*. New York: Hayworth Press, 1988.

Reed P.: Spirituality and Well Being in Terminally Ill Hospitalized Adults. *Research in Nursing and Health* 10:335, 1987.

Sanders C., ed., *The Management of Terminal Malignant Disease*. London: Edward Arnold, 1978 143-146.

Smith E., Stafanek M.E., Joseph M.V.: Spiritual Awareness, Personal Death Perspective and Psychosocial Distress Among Cancer Patients: An Initial Investigation. *Journal of Psychosocial Oncology*. 11(3): 1993, 89-102.

Sodestrom L., Martinson I.: Patients' Spiritual Coping Strategies: A Study of Nurse and Patient Perspectives. *Oncology Nursing Forum* 14(2): 41, 1987.

Turk D., Meichenbaum D., Genest M.: *Pain and Behavioural Medicine*. New York, Guilford Press, 1983.

Turk D.C. and Feldman C.S. (eds): *Non-invasive Approaches to Pain Management in the Terminally Ill*. New York: The Hayworth Press Inc. 1992.

Vachon, Mary L.S.: *Occupational Stress in the Care of the Critically Ill: Dying and the Bereaved*, NY: Hemisphere Pub. Co., 1987.

Ventafridda V., Palliative Medicine: A New Approach. *Journal of Palliative Care*, 1988.

Wasow M.: Sexuality Assessment as a Tool for Sexual Rehabilitation in Cancer Patients. *Sexuality and Disability* 5(1):28, 1982.

Weisman A.D., Worden J.W., Sobel H.J.: *Psychosocial Screening and Intervention with Cancer Patients*, Research Report. Boston: Harvard Medical School and Massachusetts General Hospital, 1980.

Wise T.: Sexuality in the Aging and Incapacitated: Disabilities and Treatment. *Psychiatric Clinics of North America* Volume 3 issue 1, 1980.

Zabora J.R., Fetting J.H., Shanley V.B. *et al.*: Predicting Conflict Among Staff Among Families of Cancer Patients During Prolonged Hospitalizations. *Journal of American Psychosocial Oncology*; 7(3): 103, 1989.

Zabora, J.R., Smith E.D.: Early Assessment and Intervention with Dysfunctional Family Systems. *Oncology* 5(2): 31, 1992.

Introduction to the Public Health Framework Exemplars

The wealth of nations depends greatly on the health of its people. As pointed out in chapter 1, health care can be thought of in terms of cure and rehabilitation OR in terms of preventing ill health. Improvements in sanitation, health education, environmental protection, improved nutrition, adequate housing conditions, relief from poverty and a general populace concerned about their own health maintenance foster optimal health status.

While social reformers in the western world of the nineteenth century attacked a number of these issues and scientific medicine attacked others, the tension between those dedicated to curing and rehabilitating those already afflicted and those dedicated to preventing illness and disease from occurring, continues to this day. The 'traditionalists' have followed a 'disease' orientation to health problems and have placed their faith in medical discoveries and new technologies. The 'nontraditionalists' have followed a philosophy that emphasises the environmental, behavioural and social science aspects of medicine which influence individual and group health status. 'Traditionalists' have given society highly specialised individualised care governed by in-depth knowledge of specific conditions, aided in diagnosis and treatment by high technology. The 'nontraditionalists' have given birth to epidemiology, biostatistics and public health programmes concerned with the overall health of communities and high risk populations within communities.

The chapter on social work in hospitals (chapter 3) explored the ways social workers have worked in a traditional medical setting. The following three chapters explore the roles, functions and possibilities for the social work profession as it exists, or might exist, with the 'nontraditionalists' working in public health and primary care settings.

Social work and public health practitioners share values and have mutual goals:

- Both are viewed as professions dedicated to the holistic promotion of physical, mental and social well-being.
- Both are based on the principle of self-determination, consumer participation and the self-improvement of those utilising their services.
- Both developed from a concern about the prevention of human deprivation and disease.

- Both use an interdisciplinary approach to problems known to have multiple causes and both employ scientific methods in solving such problems.
- Both focus on the interactive influence of inheritance, environments (human/social/physical/and man-modified), and life experience on individual and group health status.

Historical Developments in Public Health

The beginning of widespread, organised public health programmes began with the discovery of the role poor sanitation played in the spread of infectious diseases. These discoveries led to community-focused, population-based, prevention-oriented strategies designed to safeguard the public's health by minimising the spread of disease. Countries varied in their response to the public health challenge, but by the mid-1880s Britain, the USSR and the United States (among others) established locally based boards of public health. Such boards became responsible for (1) collecting vital statistics, (2) managing sanitation, (3) controlling epidemic disease by quarantine and immunisation (Burton & Smith, 1978).

The sources of data on which public health interventions were based were epidemiological studies based on incidence, prevalence and natural history; where the problem occurred; what populations were at risk; what social, environmental and medical factors were associated with the problem; and what treatment was needed when the disease or condition occurred. These methods of study are still utilised in modern public health practice.

In the social and intellectual ferment of Europe between 1860 and 1880 physicians, paid by governments to practise medicine, emerged as a professional group and formed one component of the European public health movement in Germany, France, Great Britain and other countries where health problems began to be viewed within the context of social, economic and political conditions. Russia's public physicians were closely allied to principles espoused by the German reform movement in 1850: that socio-economic conditions have an important effect on health and disease and therefore steps taken to promote health and combat disease must be social as well as medical (Krug, 1979).

While seeking to secure an important status for physicians in public health, leaders in this era were also motivated to make public health efforts a top priority in public life. This struggle was exemplified by public physicians in Russia who were members of the Pirogov Society. They resisted state-controlled medicine and promoted public health after the revolution and the Bolshevik victory (Krug, 1979).

Introduction to the Public Health Framework Exemplars

However, public health activities, preventive in nature, generally remained outside the scope of medical practice delivered for curative purposes and the treatment of those already afflicted. It was not until after the First World War that the United States, the United Kingdom and the newly formed USSR began exploring ways to integrate preventive and curative services into a holistic approach to health care, design a unified health care system, and to promote strategies to improve the health of a community as a whole (Kark, 1981).

Continuity of care, easy and equal access to care, and the importance of patient:physician relationships were concepts that were stressed in what became known as 'primary care'. The concept of primary health care includes that of a physician who (1) is locally based, (2) represents the patient's first point of contact during the course of an illness, and (3) assesses, integrates and co-ordinates the patient's needs and management throughout the course of treatment. Actions of primary care adopted by physicians may include activities designed to promote health, prevent health problems from developing, and to cure and alleviate conditions in those who are already ill or disabled.

By the 1940s the field of public health was generally recognised as the science and art of preventing disease, prolonging life and promoting health and efficiency through organised community efforts aimed at (1) sanitation of the environment; (2) control of community infections; (3) the delivery of medical and nursing service for early diagnosis and treatment of disease; (4) development of the machinery which ensured every individual in the community a standard of living adequate for the maintenance of health (Winslow, 1949).

Since the Second World War all countries have demonstrated the need for an integrated system of health care which addresses curative and individually focused care, as well as specific health needs of high-risk populations, vulnerable age-groups and the overall health of a community. South Africa pioneered with the development of community health centres and 'community oriented primary care' (Kark, 1981), and the United Kingdom developed the field of community medicine. In the United States 'family practice' and community health clinics and new types of group medical practices called Health Maintenance Organizations (HMOs) began to incorporate prevention-oriented functions within the framework of traditional medical care as a means of managing the costs of care. The World Health Organization, cognisant of the potentially positive outcomes of this work and the success of para-professional 'community health workers' in developing countries, held the first international conference on primary care at Alma Ata in the USSR in 1978 (WHO, 1978).

It is through the process of merging these two traditions — preventive and curative, institutional and community, individual and population focus — that new organisational forms may arise and present new opportunities for social work practice in relation to health.

Social Work and Public Health in the US

Social workers in the US have been employed in public health programmes since the 1920s when their participation was viewed as an extension of medical social work and they provided services to patients and families in public health programmes serving at-risk and underserved populations such as pregnant women and migrant workers. This 'casework' or 'clinical' role has expanded and now social workers in public health engage in social action, community organisation and development and social planning. Working in teams with epidemiologists, biostatisticians, physicians and nurses, social workers are valued members of public health teams both as providers of social work services, health educators, participants in the health planning process and consultants on policy matters.

The next three chapters present examples of the relationship of social work to public health and to primary care.

Chapter 5 examines the potential interface between the clinical social work role and the public health role as health care systems increasingly emphasise 'primary care' which fosters prevention and health maintenance strategies within group medical practices and co-operatives. This chapter indicates potential directions for social work practice in Russia and other European countries as the role of polyclinics change in response to changes in the priorities, funding and structure of medical care. The unique blend of public-health:curative:preventive as an orientation in out patient clinics of hospitals, polyclinics or primary care clinics funded by private fees and insurance coverage holds promise for an important public health and prevention-oriented role for social workers in medical settings which adopt a model of community-oriented primary care.

Chapter 6 deals with a public health approach to birth spacing and family planning in Russia. It emphasises Russia's historical commitment to the health of pregnant women and explores an intervention strategy utilised by a contemporary non-governmental agency operating outside the organised medical delivery system. Maternal health and its subsequent implications for the health of a society as a whole are a central function of both public health and community-oriented primary care.

Introduction to the Public Health Framework Exemplars

Chapter 7 addresses the spread of the HIV and the AIDS epidemic. The chapter stresses a public health, primary prevention perspective but also outlines the many ways social workers intervene as the affliction takes its toll on those affected by the disease process. The trajectory of the disease process and the social worker's position and responsibilities in relation to the trajectory dictate the social work role. In a situation where the social worker is attempting to prevent the spread of HIV, the social worker may be located in a public health department charged with primary prevention and may spend professional time designing, implementing and evaluating educational intervention programmes. Social workers in hospitals, outpatient clinics and group medical practices may spend their professional energies helping families and individuals cope with the shock of diagnosis, the uncertainties of treatment regimens and the patient's life course. Social workers in hospices and those providing community-based case management may deal with issues related to employment, existential crises surrounding death, and advocacy to obtain and/or retain needed services and support networks.

The chapter also serves as an illustration of the in-depth knowledge of human functioning and of disease processes that a social worker must have when working in relation to a public health problem. This is particularly true of those who serve as public policy and planning consultants and those developing intervention programmes for specialised populations.

In all three chapters the cental role and methods of preventive intervention are stressed and the prevention-oriented public health role of the social worker in modern society is examined.

References

Burton, Lloyd E. & Smith, Hugh A.; in *Public Health and Community Medicine*; 1978. Baltimore; Williams and Williams.

Kark, Sidney L.; *The Practice of Community Oriented Medicine*; 1981. New York. USA.; Appleton-Century-Crofts.

Krug, Peter Francis; *Russian Public Physicians and Revolution; The Pirogov Society, 1917 - 1920*. 1979 Ph.D. dissertation submitted to the University of Wisconsin, Madison, Wisc. USA.

Primary Health Care: *Alam Ata 1978*; WHO, Geneva, Switzerland.

Winslow, C.E.A.; 'The Evolution of Public Health and Its Objectives' in *Public Health and the World Today*; (ed) Simmonds, J. S.; 1949. Cambridge, Harvard University Press.

Chapter 5
Primary Health Care: It's Relation to Generalist Practice and to Public Health

Matthew Henk and Louise Doss Martin[1]

Introduction
Primary care is both a philosophy of care and a way of delivering health care that includes prevention of health problems, and the promotion and maintenance of positive health status as well as the diagnosis, treatment and amelioration of health problems. As a philosophy, primary care seeks to put into operation basic principles of social justice, equality, and individual responsibility for health. In this context, primary care encompasses diverse activities ranging from efforts to enhance accessibility to care, press for legislative reforms, and recognition of the role other sectors of society — such as housing, employment, education — play in health and illness (Schlesinger, 1985).

Primary care's mission is the provision of high quality, comprehensive and continuous care regardless of where a person is in the health:disease process continuum. Primary care focuses on co-ordinated, interdisciplinary provision of health care. It seeks to provide continuity of care to those being served, whether they need hospital care or care in the home and whether their condition is acute or chronic.

This chapter explores the concept of primary care and its relevance to professional social work practice. If social workers become an integral part of the staffing pattern in the primary care setting they will have an opportunity to address the psychosocial problems and contribute to the design and implementation of programmes which will not only serve individuals but also various high-risk and vulnerable populations.

The chapter presents two different roles social workers might adopt within medical organisations and settings seeking to provide primary care: (1) the generalist social work role and (2) the public health social work role. The components and implications of each role are explored.

Defining Primary Care and Primary Care Settings
Primary care organisations and settings are one component of a large, complex, and potentially intimidating medical care system. They hold an unlimited potential to improve the quality of everyday existence by focusing on health

promotion and prevention of health problems as well as on diagnosis and treatment once such problems exist.

The American Academy of Family Practice defines primary care as follows (AAFP, 1994):

> Primary Care is that care provided by physicians specifically trained for and skilled in comprehensive first contact and continuing care for persons with any undiagnosed sign, symptom, or health concern (the 'undifferentiated' patient) not limited by problem origin (biological, behavioural, or social) organ system, gender, or diagnosis.
>
> Primary Care includes health promotion, disease prevention, health maintenance, counselling, patient education, diagnosis and treatment of acute and chronic illnesses in a variety of health care settings (for example office, inpatient, critical care, long-term care, home care, day care.) Primary care is performed and managed by a personal physician, utilising other health professionals, consultation and/or referral as appropriate.
>
> Primary Care provides patient advocacy in the health care system to accomplish cost-effective care by co-ordination of health care services. Primary care promotes effective doctor:patient communication and encourages the role of the patient as a partner in health care.

A variety of authors have also defined primary care. Common denominators include:

- the setting and its providers are the first contact when an individual needs physical health, mental health or social services;
- the care provided is comprehensive and continuous: comprehensive in so far as the providers identify and treat most biological and psychosocial problems on site, and continuous in so far as the providers assume responsibility to ensure hospital and other specialised and referral services are appropriate and timely;
- care provided is affordable, geographically accessible, provides reasonable hours of access and coverage.

Most primary settings have data collection systems which can identify high-risk patient populations based on age, sex, and medical or psychosocial diagnoses. These systems help track and monitor the progress and effectiveness of treatment plans and help ensure that there is compliance with treatment regimens.

Primary Health Care: It's Relation to Generalist Practice and to Public Health

Primary care can be provided in a variety of settings. In the United States of America, these settings include:

- Federally sponsored Community Health Centres and Migrant Health Centres designed to serve urban, rural, and migrant communities that are medically underserved and critically short of physicians; goals are to provide medical services and also health promotion, mental health, nutrition, pharmaceutical, and dental services;

- Health maintenance organisations[2] and other managed care systems that are operated for profit and non-profit corporations;

- Group medical practices that are either multi-speciality or family practice, and practices of family physicians, internists, and paediatricians;

- Ambulatory or outpatient clinics of private, public, and university hospitals;

- State-, county-, and city-funded maternity and infant care, children and youth care, and primary care projects;

- Family medicine residency programmes sponsored by hospitals or universities; with services generally provided by family practice residents and faculty.

To help conceptualise the relationship between group practice, primary care, public health, and the implications for the social work role, Table I on Group Medical Practice and Primary Care illustrates similarities and differences in these settings. Suffice it to say that the boundaries between types of medical group practices and the public health orientation of such practices are very blurred at this point in the development of health care systems in many parts of the world[3].

In the discussion that follows we shall focus on the primary health care SETTING, rather than the primary care ORGANISATION, since it is in the SETTING where services are delivered.

The primary care SETTING is a PLACE where doctors and other health care professionals provide a comprehensive range of health care services which go beyond diagnostic and treatment services for specific diseases. It is a place similar to a 'one-stop shopping centre' where medical, psychological, and social problems can all be addressed.

Humanistic Approaches to Health Care: Focus on Social Work

Table I Group Medical and Primary Care

Level of Public Health Community Orientation	Group Medical Practice Model	Goals (in order of Importance)	Level of Presentation	Staffing Pattern	Unit of Focus	Method of Payment	Social Work Roles/skills
1	Traditional for profit Primary Care practices Multispeciality and Family Group Practices	Curative, but primarily acute and episodic care	Tertiary, plus some secondary or minimal health promotion/disease prevention	Internal Medicine Paediatric Family Medicine Physicians and Nurses	Individual Families	Primary, fee for services, that is, private insurance Medicare, plus self-pay	History of minimal social work involvement in these settings. Primarily psychotherapeutic
2	Contemporary primary care organisations Health Maintenance Organisations and other managed care programmes	Curative, plus some health promotion/disease prevention services	Tertiary, some secondary, some primary	Family Practice Physicians, Specialists Physicians, Social Workers Psychiatrists, Nurse Practitioners, and Physician Assistant	Individual families enrolled by contract in group medical practices called Health Maintenance Organisation	Primarily, capitation, that is, annual flat rate payment per patient per year which is paid by the employer	Psychotherapeutic, behaviour modification, team and collaborative skills, education and teaching skills, group work skills, case-work skills and family therapy skills
3	Federally funded community and migrant health centres, county and city clinics and other comprehensive non-profit clinics	Comprehensive services which focus on individuals, families, and the environment. Interactions are designed to promote health of individuals, groups and the community. Health promotion and disease prevention are key elements. Linkages with local community resources such as community mental health	Primary, Secondary, Tertiary	Community Health Nurses, Physician Assistant and Nurse Practitioners, community Health Workers, Psychologists, Health Educators and Dentists	Individuals and Families. Community as defined by geographic area. Total environment, high-risk, and underserved populations (for example, homeless, refugees, unwed mothers, migrants, and HIV)	Primarily Medicaid (indigent), Medicare, and patients who have no resources	Psychotherapeutic, team and collaborative skills, group work skills, case-work, and family therapy skills, data analysis and public health skills, survey research skills, policy analysis and development skills, planning and evaluation skills

Primary Health Care: It's Relation to Generalist Practice and to Public Health

The primary care ORGANISATION is a FORMAL ORGANISATION of health care professionals, brought together on a contractual basis, for the purpose of providing comprehensive services to people who contract with the organisation to obtain health care. Costs for these services are paid by a combination of fees charged directly to patients and their families, fees charged to and paid for by the patient's insurance company, or in some instances by federal, state or local programmes funded by the government.

Medical organisations that provide primary care have an explicit or implicit contract between those who provide care and the patients who seek care. This contract dictates that providers of care will assume major responsibility to preserve and to improve the health of the people they serve. This contract, or understanding, between the consumers of service and the providers of service means that the primary care organisation, in its setting, is able to address a wide range of problem areas, be they biological, personal, familial, or environmental.

As a result of this relationship, providers in a primary care setting may initiate contacts with a patient prior to a patient's request for services. For example, to write to elderly patients offering to provide flu shots or to parents offering to provide immunisations to children, or to offer parent effectiveness classes.

In this arena of primary care, administrators and physicians struggle to decide if the social worker should function primarily as a 'generalist' or a 'specialist'. The social worker participates in this decision by carefully analysing both the organisation's expectations and patient needs before committing to specific roles such as advocate, therapist, or public health social worker. For example, if the administration decides that the mental health therapist's role will be the most important, the social worker could be fully scheduled with patients within several months and have no time to serve new patients, much less to serve patients who need help with social and environmental problems. Similarly, if the public health role or advocacy role is selected, some patients' mental health problems would ultimately not be addressed.

The following sections will define the generalist's role and the public health role and how they can best be integrated into the primary care setting.

The Generalist's Role
The variety and complexity of primary care settings and the diversity of demands made upon social workers practising in them create a need for a versatile social work practice model. Schlesinger (1985) points out that primary care provides a unique opportunity to practise in a manner congruent with social work's traditional

mandate *to address both individual needs and deficits in the larger social environment.* She also notes that such an approach can generate excitement and respect for the social worker's role. The generalist's approach, which requires that the social worker examine a problem from a broad perspective and be prepared to intervene at multiple levels in a range of situations, provides a suitable framework for such practice (Sheafor & Landon, 1987). This section discusses a methodology for setting social work priorities, identifies the key components of the generalist role, and presents guidelines for establishing this role in a primary care setting.

Defining the Generalist Social Worker Role and Setting Priorities
Specifics of the generalist model of social work practice are outlined in chapter 1. The following discussion relates this model specifically to primary care settings.

Primary care social workers practise in a variety of settings that differ in locale, populations served, and major functions. Schlesinger (1985) points out, however, that certain features are characteristic of social work practice in any health care setting:

- Social work services are often viewed as ancillary to the major function of the setting;
- Patients are often seen during a crisis situation;
- Primary care settings are complex organisations;
- When specialised services are offered within primary care, most social work providers must develop the relevant expertise needed to provide them;
- When a diverse population is served, most workers need to become familiar with a variety of physical and mental disorders;
- Opportunities for prevention and health promotion must be recognised and used when primary health care is delivered as part of another service system, such as the work-place or school;
- Outreach and health planning require knowledge of community health problems and priorities.

Thus, it is critical that primary care social workers be aware of (1) the organisational structure and major functions of the setting; (2) the recurrent medical, psychological, and social problems exhibited in the patient population and the community, (3) current health, and social policy developments and regulations; and (4) their own areas of expertise and limitations (Schlesinger, 1985).

Primary Health Care: It's Relation to Generalist Practice and to Public Health

Optimally, the social work role is defined and a social service plan is established for the setting prior to the introduction of social work services or the addition of new social work staff. Ultimately, the roles for social workers should be based upon criteria that have been mutually agreed upon by the organisation, those who are the providers of service within that organisation, and the social worker. No single social worker can meet the needs of all patients, providers, and administrators, but if expectations are clarified and priorities are set, role conflict can be minimised, dissatisfaction and inter-staff conflicts that could detract from patient care can be minimised.

The first step in setting priorities for social work activities in the primary care setting is to assess the significant health and psychosocial needs of the patient population served. This can be done by using existing data or by administering patient and/or provider questionnaires or by initiating appropriate ongoing data collection procedures.

The second step is to meet with administrators and determine their goals in light of the problems that have been identified by an assessment of patient needs. It is essential that the primary care social worker has a clear understanding of the needs and expectations of the setting in order to determine the extent to which each aspect of the generalist role should be used.

Essential Components: the Generalist Perspective

Primary care requires a practice approach that considers the entire situation when making an assessment and when planning and implementing intervention. Assessment and goal-setting cannot be limited by the way a problem is initially presented because *the presenting problem in the primary care setting often is not the true problem, but rather one that has been medicalised.* In primary care settings, the social worker's interventions cannot be constrained by a worker's methodological bias.

The primary care social worker has been described as a generalist with a broad knowledge base and the broad repertoire of skills that are needed because health problems have multiple causes. As pointed out in chapter 1, generalist practice assumes that the worker has an eclectic theoretical base, uses a systems framework for assessment, is oriented to multilevel interventions, and takes responsibility for guiding the problem-solving or planned change process. The social work process in generalist practice includes intake and engagement, assessment, planning and contracting, intervention, monitoring and evaluation, and termination (Sheafor & Landon, 1987).

The Generalist Process:
Intake, Engagement and Assessment with Patients and Families

In these phases, the social worker makes contact with the patient or family, identifies the issues to be addressed, determines whether service can be provided or if referral to other services should be made, initiates the helping relationship, engages the patient in the planned change or problem-solving process, and collects and analyses factual and impressionistic data concerning the patient and family systems and the other systems involved (Sheafor & Landon, 1987). The primary care setting and procedure determine the point at which patient and social worker meet. In some settings all new patients are referred to the social worker for psychological assessment. In other settings, patients are identified by social workers through the use of high-risk screening criteria, or they may be referred to the social worker by physicians (Miller, 1987).

Using the epidemiologic concept of 'risk' is critical to identifying patients and families who need social work intervention. Risk factors are biological, psychological, social, demographic or cultural characteristics that increase the vulnerability of a patient or population to various health or mental health problems. Table II is an example of criteria that can be used to identify women at risk of miscarriages and other pregnancy difficulties.

TABLE II
Maternal, Medical, Reproductive and Social Risk Factors
Medical and Reproductive Risk Factors

- Chronic hypertension
- Renal disease
- Diabetes mellitus
- Cardiac arrest
- Cancer
- Sickle-cell trait ot disease
- Anaemia
- Thyroid disorder
- Gastrointestinal or liver disease
- Epilepsy
- Recurrent urinary tract infection
- Nutritional deficiency
- Mental retardation
- Psychiatric disorder
- Drug addiction, alcoholism or heavy drinking
- Two or more spontaneus or induced abortions
- Previous stillbirth or neonatal death
- Previous premature delivery, low birth weight or intrauterine retardation
- Previously excessively large infant
- Fifth or greater pregnancy
- Previous Rh isoimmunisation
- Pre-eclampsia
- Previous infant with hereditary disorder or congenitial anomaly
- Previous infant birth-damaged or required neonatal intensive care
- Family history of hereditary disorder
- Maternal age under 18 or over 35

Table II (cont'd)
Social Risk Factors

- Poverty
- Substandard housing or environment
- . Lack of transportation
- Less than high school education
- Member of oppressed or under-served minority group
- Single mother
- Accidental or unwanted pregnancy
- Adolescent pregnancy
- Lack of experience in infant and child care
- Social isolation
- Stressful life event or conditions
- Marital conflict
- Family conflict
- History of child abuse or neglect
- Drug or alcohol addiction

Depending on the primary care setting, social risk criteria can be incorporated into the initial assessment of all new patients, can be used by the social worker for high-risk screening through record review, or can be used by the physician or other providers as the basis for referral to social work. The 'Public Health Role' section provides further information on case finding, outreach, and programme development that flows from the identification of high risk groups. In addition to helping identify patients and families in need of service, high risk factor screening can assist the social worker in determining whether to provide the services needed, whether referral is indicated, and which issues should be addressed by social work intervention within the setting.

Generalist Process:
Planning, Contracting and Intervening with Patients and Families

Once an assessment has been made and problems or risk factors have been identified, the generalist social worker, in consultation with the primary care physician and other relevant providers: (1) considers with the patient or family the range of solutions available and the advantages and disadvantages of each; 2) selects the most acceptable option; and (3) develops a formal or informal health care plan designating responsibilities for each party involved.

During intervention, each of the systems involved carries out the agreed upon responsibility (Sheafor & Landon, 1987). *Effective use of skills in consultation and ongoing interdisciplinary collaboration are crucial* to the successful planning and implementation intervention. The continuous care responsibility of primary care does not mean that a single provider or programme directly undertakes all activities necessary to resolve or ameliorate a patient's problems. It does mean, however, that the primary care setting takes responsibility for ensuring that all of the various actions needed to accomplish the mutually agreed upon health care plan are taken.

Time and technical capability are critical determinants of the nature and extent of the generalist social worker's involvement. Thus, significant activities include: assisting patients in obtaining community resources, referral to other agencies, and advocacy on behalf of patients or patient groups. The ability to link people with those particular sources of help appropriate to their needs is fundamental to all social work practise. In the clinical situation, a primary care user/patient/consumer may require a variety of social services. Advocacy skills may be needed to engage another organisation's commitment to providing a necessary service to a patient.

Another way social workers utilise community resources is by networking and linking patients with self-help and mutual aid groups and by generating resources within patients' existing social networks. For example, adult children and neighbours might be organised to identify a mutually agreeable contribution to a disabled person's well-being. As an example, a terminally ill cancer patient was able to remain at home rather than be placed in a nursing home because a social worker helped the patient's elderly husband ask a neighbour friend who was a retired nurse to assist with the injection of pain medication.

In addition to helping individual patients use existing resources, generalist social workers may seek to remedy resource deficits by changes in their own primary care programmes. For example, one family practise setting observed the various health problems associated with death of a spouse and initiated specific services directed to all the recently widowed persons who were enrolled in their services.

Primary care settings serving the poor often serve populations of cultural and ethnic diversity. Social workers play an active role in developing programmes that are sensitive to the health beliefs and behaviours of various ethnic groups (Schlesinger, 1985). Programme consultation and advocacy skills can facilitate accomplishing such objectives.

Expertise in linking patients with formal and informal community resources and in improving the content and quality of care in existing programmes constitutes core generalist practise components. Creativity and innovation are also required if patients' needs are to be met.

Generalist Role in Development of Community Services and Social Policy Change

The primary care social worker practising from the generalist perspective *must go beyond clinical problem solving*. Resource deficits become a concern not only to those patients already requiring treatment or rehabilitation but also to those at risk. As discussed further in the Public Health section, social workers can use data collection systems to identify high-risk populations and to design and implement preventive interventions.

In addition, the primary care social worker can (1) identify community agencies accountable for specific high-risk populations, (2) negotiate service agreements between primary care programmes and other community programmes, and (3) advocate for needed services (Schlesinger, 1985). For example, a primary care social worker seeing substantial numbers of pregnant teens in a community where schools do not offer family life and sex education can initiate and/or join a community-based planning or advocacy group sharing this concern. The goal in such a situation would be to bring about comprehensive and effective school programmes with potential for reducing the community-wide incidence of unintended teen pregnancy.

On a broader scale, social workers in primary care should be alert to patient problems that result from inadequate and inequitable public policy. Social workers should take the lead in building coalitions, setting policy, undertaking relevant research, and administering programmes to resolve disparities in health status (Gitterman, Black & Stein, 1985). This means providing clinical services to help overcome cultural and economic barriers to the access and utilisation of clinical services. It also requires using knowledge of macro levels of intervention to develop data and disseminate information and to influence public policy (Siefert, 1988).

The primary care social worker must understand general strategies for creating change: (1) developing new information about a problem and making it available to those who need or are receptive to it; (2) educating and stimulating the public; and (3) using direct administrative or political power or control to change services, systems or programmes (Torrens, 1978).

Primary care social workers must know the basic steps required to carry out a strategy for change: (1) accurately assess need, (2) carefully establish objectives, (3) obtain and review relevant and supportive data, and (4) identify those people and groups with the power to accomplish change. The need for political action and advocacy has never been greater. Action to improve social conditions is part of the social worker's professional responsibility in whatever setting they practise.

Generalist: Monitoring and Evaluation
For the primary care social worker practising from the generalist perspective, monitoring and evaluation are conducted throughout the change process. This helps ascertain the success of the planned intervention and the possibility of using other methods to achieve desired outcomes (Sheafor & Landon, 1987). Interdisciplinary collaboration permits monitoring of the patient's movement at every level of care.

Intervention may be evaluated in terms of process, effect, and outcome: Process evaluation monitors the acceptability or quality of practise. Effect evaluation focuses on the immediate effect or the intervention on the short-term goals of intervention. Outcome evaluation measures the long-term health and social benefits of intervention in terms of mortality, morbidity, and overall cost-effectiveness (Green, Kreuter, Deeds, & Partridge, 1980). Different designs may be used in evaluation, ranging from the collection of routine data on an ongoing basis to full-scale evaluation research projects (Siefert, 1988).

In summary, a decision has to be made as to what proportion of clinical or programmematic services are to be provided by the social worker. The following section on the Public Health Role is described in detail to assist in that decision-making process.

Public Health Social Work Role
Social work — with its historical commitment to vulnerable and oppressed populations, its dual focus on person and situation, and its commitment to social action on behalf of the under served — shares considerable ground with public health (Siefert, 1986). This is especially true in light of a definition of public health as a social movement concerned with protecting and promoting the collective health of the community.

Public health social work should not be defined by the SETTING in which one practises but by HOW ONE PRACTISES in the setting. The public health social work role, unlike the advocacy, brokerage, or therapist role, begins the intervention process by assessing the collective patient population rather than by assessing individual patient's needs.

The primary care setting has some unique characteristics which allow for the development of a public health social work practise. They include:

- a commitment to the concepts of health promotion and disease prevention;
- a willingness to assume the responsibility to provide comprehensive care; this requires multi-focused interventions by a variety of health professionals;
- data collection systems that will identify high-risk patients;
- a radically different contract between provider and patient that allows the provider to intervene with the patient before the onset of illness and before services are initiated by the patient;
- physician providers who are trained to address both biomedical and psychosocial problems;
- a specific and finite target population that can be identified and treated in a rational, organised fashion.

The public health role is significantly different from the generalist role described earlier in the chapter as it does not focus on a specific intervention for a specific patient at a specific stage of the disease process. Rather, it requires many interventions for both the patient and environment, throughout the disease process continuum.

The public health social worker should develop a variety of interventions, for both the patient and his environment, throughout the health:illness continuum.

This role requires considerable discipline and the ability to follow a rigorous problem-solving process. The process requires a knowledge of data and data collection systems as well as the skill to organise programmes that will result in concrete and specific outcomes.

Such a prescriptive process is necessary not only to measure outcomes but also to measure cost effectiveness and to set standards for acceptable practise and to insure professional accountability.

Consideration for developing a public health practise within primary care settings evolves from collaboration between decision-makers and social workers within the primary care organisation. Two positive aspects are: (1) care can be provided more efficiently and effectively and (2) the biomedical and psychosocial problems encountered in the primary care setting are so numerous that they cannot be addressed on an individual basis.

Public health social work practise could be developed in a primary care setting using a five-phase problem-solving process:

- Assessment of needs
- Targeting interventions
- Prioritising interventions
- Planning intervention strategies
- Evaluating the effectiveness of the interventions.

Examples of this process will be provided later in this section.

Public Health Process: Assessment
Assessment requires information or data. Primary care settings in the United States of America have manual and computerised data systems which allow for easy identification of patients by age, sex, and medical and psychosocial diagnosis. Analysis of these data is the first step in the process of developing and prioritising intervention programmes for patients at risk.

Since specific and comprehensive data on patients are usually available in most primary care settings, high-risk patients can be easily identified. The questions: Who are the teenage diabetics? Who are the pregnant mothers who smoke, drink, or abuse drugs? Which young children reside in older homes with high concentrations of lead can usually be answered. With recent advances in computer technology, patients at risk can be identified in minutes.

Public Health Process: Interventions

Several authors have used matrices to identify targets of intervention for public health problems (Haddon, 1980; Margolis & Runyan, 1983). Such matrices allow public health practitioners and their settings to view interventions in their totalities and not just in relationship to an acute phase of a biological problem.

Knowing *when and where* interventions can occur for any given problem is essential in the development of a model matrix for public health interventions.

When. Because the disease moves along a continuum, it is important to know when a health promotion or disease prevention programme should be developed. The 'when' could be viewed in primary, secondary, and tertiary terms:

Primary Prevention includes activities undertaken to prevent the occurrence of disease. Examples include health education, encouraging the use of condoms to prevent AIDS, immunisations, and parent effectiveness classes.

Secondary Prevention includes activities undertaken to intervene after disease can be detected but before it is symptomatic. Examples are screening for lead levels, hypertension, cholesterol, and high-risk factors for child abuse, alcohol abuse and AIDS.

Tertiary Prevention includes activities undertaken to prevent the progression of symptomatic disease. This includes the development and implementation of treatment programmes for patients with common diagnoses, such as diet workshops for obese patients.

Where. The other component of the matrix identifies where the intervention will take place, that is, biological, individual/family, and environment. Biological includes molecule, cell, tissue, organ, or nervous system. Individual/family includes the patient, spouse, nuclear family, and extended family. Environment includes neighbourhood, community, church, school, and government.

This matrix is illustrated in Table III with the prevention of infant mortality/morbidity as the problem. This type of matrix allows the care providers to view all the targets of intervention and also allows each health professional to clarify their role in solving the specific problem.

Table III   Prevention of Infant Mortality/Morbidity

WHEN	BIOLOGICAL	INDIVIDUAL/ FAMILIES	ENVIRONMENT
PRIMARY PREVENTION	To ensure that adequate and accessible comprehensive health services, including adequate nutrition and family planning, are available to all women age 15-45	Educating young women to utilise preventive health services so they are in optimal health prior to pregnancy	Develop comprehensive women's health services at local, regional and national levels. Assist women to prevent unintended pregnancies by ensuring availability of a range of birth control methods to improve women's health. Support development of non-governmental organisation and advocacy groups
SECONDARY PREVENTION	To provide pregnancy testing and early identification of pregnancy classes. Due to prevalence of faetal alcohol syndrome, there is a critical need to institute alcohol treatment programmes	Initiation of preventive care, testing and early certification of pregnancy. Childbirth education counselling and classes, including smoking cessation and alcohol and drug treatment groups.	Identifying women in first trimester who have high risk behaviours detrimental to their health and that of their foetus (for example, smoking or alcohol)
TERTIARY PREVENTION	To ensure optimal care to all infants born at low birth weight or infants with or at high risk of development disability. High quality paediatric care for well babies.	Post-partum care for mothers, including assessment and care and availability of birth control. Ongoing paediatric care and assessment for early detection of diseases. Immunisation for babies	Development of neo-natal intensive care facilities for low birth weight infants and other high risk infants.

In addition to these efforts, it is essential that the power that is inherently associated with physicians and group practises be used to create change in legislation and institutional policies to better meet the needs of patients. The source of power relates primarily to the status of physicians or the group practise. The number of patients also represents a significant power base when lobbying for various changes. Social workers need to mobilise this power when they lobby for social change when necessary. They also need to use this power base to ensure that legislation and policy positions do not adversely affect a specific population group.

To this end, the social worker must be able to develop coalitions, consortia, committees, and associations to assist in this effort.

Public Health Process: Prioritising Interventions

Presently, most decisions regarding the development of health promotion/disease prevention programmes in primary care settings are subjective and arbitrary. To organise the process, the public health social worker must assist providers and administrators to agree on broad goals and specific interventions. The importance of this process cannot be overstated.

Interventions should:

- Meet the goals and objectives established by the setting;
- Address mortality/ morbidity issues of the practise;
- Be inexpensive and realistic;
- Improve the health status of a significant number of patients.

For example, if one of the setting's goals is to improve the health status of the elderly and if a significant number of elderly were diagnosed as having had the flu during the previous year, then providing flu shots would be a high priority. Data in the age/sex registry would be available to identify the risk group, and existing staff should be available to develop and implement the outreach effort. Cost would be minimal, and the immunisations, known to be effective, would have a positive effect on the health of patients. It would also be cost-effective since the cost of care for one patient who is hospitalised with complications from the flu could pay for the total outreach effort.

Public Health Process: Planning Intervention Strategies

Once a problem is identified and an intervention is agreed upon, a plan needs to be designed. A work planning process is needed to set objectives that are specific, time-phased, and measurable. Responsibility must also be assigned to individuals and agencies to carry out specific tasks.

Each objective should relate to the broad goals agreed upon by the decision makers of the setting. Using the flu immunisation outreach as an example, the objective might read: 'To immunise 90 per cent of all patients over 65 years of age.' Actions to be taken are often grouped according to levels, or steps. Each "step" should identify each activity that must be accomplished to meet the objective. Individuals are assigned responsibility to accomplish each activity within a specific time frame. Actions might include:

- Obtaining the names and addresses of each patient over the age of 65.
- Writing letters informing patients when and where they can be immunised.
- Obtaining the inoculation from the city or state health department.
- Assigning responsibilities to nursing staff to inoculate patients.
- Mobilising community resources to assist in patient transportation if necessary.
- Setting up planning meetings to determine if immunisation should be given during regular working hours, or on specific days during the week, or during evening hours.

Once again, a carefully laid out work plan will identify each step that needs to be taken to achieve the objective. Developing a written plan will also encourage the staff members to be accountable for their contributions in meeting the objective.

Tasks may be assigned to any member of the multidisciplinary staff — nurses, physicians or administrators.

Public Health Evaluation

There is a tradition in public health in regard to specificity of targets and goals, accountability in terms of cost-effectiveness, and concrete evidence that interventions produce the anticipated results. Undoubtedly this stems from the objectivity demanded by epidemiologists and biostatisticians to which public health staff must become accustomed. Part of this process is referred to as 'management by objectives'. This involves an organisational planning process which involves staff in the development of organisational goals and objectives and the measurement of the degree to which objectives have been achieved.

In a situation where specific objectives are set but not met, a good work planning process which specifies tasks, completion dates, and completed reporting on results and outcomes, permits the social worker to determine where the process failed. New plans can then be developed for subsequent efforts to improve the health promotion/disease prevention programme.

Evaluation can be viewed in terms of process and health status outcomes. Process outcomes are evaluated by measuring the success of each step required to meet the objective. Health status outcomes are evaluated by measuring the degree to which the patient's health improved.

An effective work planning process helps identify deficiencies in the system and the individuals or agencies that failed to meet their responsibilities. Well-developed work plans also go further than evaluating process outcomes because the real objective is to improve the health status of the patients. The establishment of a quality assurance committee within the organisation, comprising key staff and personnel, is often a useful option to evaluate such work plans (Henk, 1989).

Conclusion

Social workers have an important and vital role to play in primary care settings, particularly since such settings are viewed as 'one-stop shopping centres' that can address a variety of physical, psychological, social and environmental problems. Those providing primary care are in an ideal position to aggressively intervene in patients' lives at the earliest stage of the problem-solving process. Social workers must capitalise on this setting and provide leadership in the development of interventions to serve primary care patients and populations and emphasise preventive services. Social workers can meet the needs of a significant number of patients but, more importantly, the primary care setting can be utilised to create positive social change, develop public policies, and address a variety of social justice issues.

Notes

1. This chapter was written in the authors' private capacity. No official support or endorsement by the Department of Health and Human Services or Public Health Service should be inferred.
2. 'Medical co-operative' is the Russian term most similar to the concept of health maintenance organisation. In Britain 'GP Fundholder' is the most applicable term.
3. Revision of the National Health Service in Britain has led to increased awareness of the role of primary care in relation to community care. See for example Pietroni, P. and Pietroni, C. (1996).

References

AAFP Official Definition of Primary Care. (1994). Kansas City, MO: AAFP Reprint 302.

Campbell, Joseph. (1988). *The power of myth* [Series with Bill Moyers]. PBS TV. New York; Doubleday.

Dana, B. (1983). Collaboration in primary care, or is it? In R.S. Miller (Ed.), *Primary health care: More than medicine.*Englewood Cliffs, NJ: Prentice-Hall.

Ell, K., & Morrison, D.R. (1981). *Primary care. Health and Social Work,* 6(4), Supplement, 35S-48S.

Froom, J., Culpepper, L. & Boisseau, V. (1977). An integrated medical record and data system for primary care, III. The diagnostic index — manual and computer methods and applications. *Journal of Family Practises,* 5, 113-120.

Gitterman, A., Black, R. & Stein, F. (1985). *Public health social work in maternal and child health: A forward plan.* Rockville, MD: Maternal and Child Health, US Department of Health and Human Services.

Green, L.W., Kreuter, M.W., Deeds, S.G., & Partridge, K.B. (1980)*Health education planning: A diagnostic approach.* Palo Alto, CA: Mayfield.

Haddon, W. (1980). Advance of the epidemiology of injury as a basis for public policy. *Public Health Report,* 95, 411-421.

Henk, M. (1989). *Social Work in Primary Care* Sage; California.

Margolis, L.H. & Runyan, C.W. (1983). Accidental policy: An analysis of the problem of unintended injuries of childhood. *American Journal of Orthopsychiatry,* 53, 629-643.

Miller, R.S. (1987). Primary health care. *Encyclopedia of social work.* Silver Spring, MD: National Association of Social Workers.

Pietroni, P. and Pietroni C. *Innovation in Community Care and Primary Health* (1996) Churchill Livingstone, London.

Public Health Service, Department of Health, Education & Welfare (1975), September. *Work plan manual.* Kansas City, MO: Public Health Service.

Renner, John. (1977). Academic missions of family medicine. In T.E. Bryan (Ed.), *Fogarty International Centre proceedings*. Washington, DC: DHEW Publications No. (NIH) 77-1062.

Schlesinger, E.G. (1985). *Health care social work practice: Concepts and strategies*. St Louis: Times Mirror/Mosby.

Sheafor, B.W., & Landon, P.S. (1987). Generalist perspective. *Encyclopedia of social work*. Silver Spring, MD: National Association of Social Workers.

Siefert, K. (1985). Identifying mothers at medical and social risk. In D. Rodman & A. Murphy (Eds.), *Perinatal care in the '80's: Social work strategies for prevention and intervention*. Rockville, MD: Maternal and Child Health, US Department of Health and Human Services.

Siefert, K (1986). 'Theoretical Base for Social Work Interventions' in Elizabeth Watkins (ed) *Infant Mortality, Morbidity and Childhood Handicapping Conditions: Bio-psychosocial Factors* Bureau of Health Care Delivery and Assistance, DHHS, Rockville, Md.

Siefert, K. (1988). Disparity in birth outcomes: Implications for public health social work. In J. Morton (Ed.). *Advocacy and outreach: Developing social work program to prevent low birthweight and infant mortality*. Rockville, MD: Maternal and Child Health, US Department of Health and Human Services.

Torrens, P. (1978). *The American health care system: Issues and problems*. St Louis, MO: Mosby.

US Department of Health and Human Services. (1980). *Programme management: A guide for improving program decisions*. Atlanta, GA: Centres for Disease Control.

Chapter 6
Social Work and Family Planning in Russia: A Public Health Perspective

Natalia Grigorieva

Introduction

In order to solve the many social problems in our society, clarification of the roles, functions and mechanisms of social work, especially in the health protection area, becomes increasingly important.

Many people, acknowledging the primary importance of preserving women's and children's health as society's task, propose a social work profession mostly connected to the activities and associations of the medical profession. However, the preservation of women's and children's health requires a variety of social services and social work programmes within national, regional and local governments which are created both to assist the medical profession AND to provide opportunities for social work to address health-related concerns in the social service domain.

Planned parenthood has been identified by the United Nations as a human right. Planned parenthood programmes, in conjunction with other social and economic projects, appear to be a major aspect of successful social development programmes. The quality of people's lives and well-being may be drastically changed by providing free access to information and services in the area of birth control. This requires medical, clinical, and social services which create for women conditions that are: (1) conducive to communicating their concerns, (2) provide access to reference books, and (3) create opportunities to exchange opinions about health, anxieties, doubts and demands. This means that social workers must provide direct help to clients in medical settings and also provide activities *outside* medical settings which can help clients take a first step in thinking about their own health.

A factor common to all planned parenthood programmes is CHOICE. The right to choose means, first of all, access to information. Any woman, or any man, has a right to choice of contraceptive methods and therefore has the right to know about all existing methods. However, when no information on contraception is available or access to options regarding contraceptive measures is limited, where no special structures exist to support men and women who wish to discuss and find a solution to their own reproductive problems, there is an absence of contraceptive choice.

This chapter explores the historical developments in Russia which have affected the well-being of pregnant mothers and children. These developments move from concern about the care of foundlings and about protecting mothers and children during the birth process, to modern-day family planning as a means of protecting the well-being of mothers and children.

The History of Charity in Medical Birth-assisting Services

The system of help for mothers and children has its own history in Russia. Russians can say that social work in the medical area, as it is called today, historically was mainly connected with charity activity.

The most widely recognised form of providing assistance to those who needed it in Russia was a blend of public care which had its own structure, motivation and goals. Public care, as organised by the great Princes, the Tsar and the Church, provided different types of aid to the poor and orphans. As early as the eleventh century there were shelters for the poor and homeless, hospitals for the diseased and disabled, orphanages for children. Donors included state and departmental organisations as well as private donors and public charitable entities. Motivation for such care and concern was civic solidarity and a societal concern for poor people's welfare.

By the fourteenth century, two directions were more clearly established in the development of care for the public. The first direction was the continuation of the tradition of Kiev's Russian princes who demonstrated the giving of individual charity to beggars, the sick and the orphaned. The second direction could be characterised as a reinforcement of the organisational basis for services and elaboration of the forms and the scale of state public care. However, as social problems expanded in scope and complexity, new approaches were needed that would not be restricted either by private charity or the existing the forms of church and monastery charity.

The first step in creating a state administration for public care in Russia was an order to the country's Patriarch Department, and later to the newly organised Pharmacology Department, to implement this important activity. The concept of a structured system of public care was initiated during the reign of Feodor Alexeevich who, in 1682, issued a decree to build hospitals and nursing homes in Moscow. This decree for the first time demonstrated measures to fight the 'social evil' known as professional begging.

The organisation for management of the emerging public care system began during the reign of Peter the Great. The main basics of the system established by Peter I were further developed during the reign of Elizabeth Petrovna (1741-1761). She was eager to maintain and enhance the benefits of the public care structure. For the first time public care homes were established and they served widows and daughters of honoured officials.

The greatest impact on the public care system was made by Catherine II. During her reign, in 1775, she issued the 'Decree Institution to Administrative Provinces'. This decree established a system of public care for 'all civic estates' by legislative decree. Special Public Care Departments under the rule of a governor were stipulated for every province. The responsibilities of these departments included establishing and maintaining public schools, orphan homes, hospitals, pharmacies, nursing homes, homes for the incurably diseased, workhouses and mental hospitals.

To finance the foundation and maintenance of all these institutions, every Public Care Department received 15,000 roubles from the state treasury as initial capital. They were granted permission to increase this amount by giving interest loans to individuals and by accepting private contributions. Moreover, permission was granted to cities, communities, villages and private individuals to establish any of these useful institutions on their own initiative, and a 'Municipal Decree' published in 1785 permitted municipalities to allot part of their means to public care departments.

Between 1810 and 1819 the Ministry of Police was in charge of public medical care, and public care departments were managed by a division of the Internal Affairs Department. The Ministry of Police also included the Medical Department itself. In addition, a Medical Council was organised, consisting of officials from other structures not subordinated to the Ministry of Police. In 1819, the Ministry of Police was united with the Ministry of Internal Affairs. However, all existing structures, almost without changes, were left untouched. No measures regarding medical affairs in Russia could be presented for the Tsar's approval without permission of the Medical Council, which was controlled by the Ministry of Police. Later, during the reign of Paul I, medical boards consisting of surgeon, obstetrician and obligatory inspector, were organised in every province. Hospitals in villages were an option depending on a landlord's good will.

In 1852 Public Health Committees were established in provinces and administrative centres. They included honourable representatives of a city's administration and representatives of the city's population. Reform legislation in 1864, placed all issues of medical and sanitation matters under authority of new Zemsky (district) Institutions, and Public Care Departments were abolished. Until the middle of the

1860s a system of somewhat regulated medical care existed almost exclusively in cities. One of the most important tasks for Zemstva (districts) was establishing rural medical care. By 1880, 292 medical consultation offices were opened in various villages and 34 Zemsky (district) provinces. They provided distribution of medicine and medical care free of charge. There were also nine Zemsky provinces at this time and the Public Care Department Medical Institution System remained in existence in those provinces. One of Zemstvos (district) activity areas was training doctors' assistants and obstetricians on site.

By the beginning of the twentieth century, the organisation of medical and obstetrical help was insignificant. Province hospitals and hospitals in some cities had special maternity divisions, but rural populations seldom used these facilities. It was not until 1889 that women doctors were granted the right to hold positions in foundling institutions and gained the right to manage Zemsky medical districts and medical institutions. In 1898 the Tsar approved a Ministry of Internal Affairs' Decree allowing women to become Civil Servants.

In spite of all these reorganisations, a system of obstetric help for the entire population did not exist. Toward the end of the last century some Zemstva invited a few women obstetricians to undertake a special mission. They were to '. . . distribute medical information, to gather midwives in every village and to give them advice on how to handle recently confined women, to provide financial help to diseased and to talk with healthy patients . . .'. This was an important beginning.

The Nobility Establish Their Own Charities

The nobility also undertook to establish their own charitable societies in Russia. The first of these, the Foundling Institution of Noble Girls, was founded by Catherine II in 1764 and was initiated by special by-law. In his Special Decree of 12 November, 1796, Paul I appointed his wife Maria Feodorovna to put great efforts into development of a system of public care in Russia and to 'manage the Foundling Society'. In 1854 all of the approximately 60 organisations were united under the common name of 'Administration of Empress Maria's Institutions'. In 1870 most hospitals, including the large Foundling Homes in St Petersburg and Moscow, were removed from the authority of Empress Maria's Institutions and transferred to the jurisdiction of municipal authorities.

One of the most important tasks of foundling homes, besides caring for children of unmarried women, was providing care for 'poor mothers not only of unknown status but also legal'. Returning from a trip abroad, it was County Betzkoy who suggested that Catherine II establish in Russia institutions in which 'poor pregnant women would find shelter and help, and which would save newly born

Social Work and Family Planning in Russia: A Public Health Perspective

babies from death and this way will bring more benefits for the state'. It was in April 1764 that pregnant women were first admitted to the maternity home of the Moscow Foundling Home.

Originally, this hospital was founded in secret. It accepted only 'illegal' pregnant women from both the common people and the nobility. There was a secret branch for common women and a special branch for nobility. Both programmes worked on the principles of strict anonymity and confidentiality. The maternity home was financed partly by charity donations and partly by the state. It received food and clothing as donations. Many married women, aware of the good conditions, expressed a desire to deliver babies in the hospital. An offical maternity hospital was opened in 1805 to meet these requests. The medical personnel for both hospitals was the same.

During 36 years of Maria Feodorovna's consortship 16,876 women delivered babies in this maternity hospital and 5,876 illegitimate children were born and stayed in the foundling home. By the beginning of the twentieth century, the staff in Moscow hospital consisted of the chief doctor, the doctor obstetrician and four women obstetrician assistants.

As already noted, foundling homes for orphans and/or abandoned children existed in Russia as early as the eleventh century. Maternity hospitals were created in the 1700s and were connected to the foundling homes. In a further advancement of services to pregnant women, midwife institutes emerged. In 1880 the Midwife Institute in Moscow was opened under the auspices of the Moscow Foundling Home. Grown-up residents of the foundling home entered this institute to study midwife skills and later to provide home birthing services in the various cities of the Empire and, in complicated cases, to advise women to go to the hospital. In 1870, a special clinic of gynaecological diseases was opened.

In St Petersburg, a Foundling Home opened in 1772, with the same structure as the one operating in Moscow. In 1835 the St Petersburg Delivery Assistance Institution was opened on the site of the Maternity Hospital. A Midwife Institute and a faculty for rural midwives, located in Kalinkinskaya Hospital, was a part of the Delivery Assistance Institute. This institute also later became a special college for training obstetricians.

By the beginning of the twentieth century, huge amounts of capital were needed to finance all kinds of social assistance implemented by these public care institutions. Common efforts of the state, charitable organisations and the institutions themselves, raised almost 405 million roubles, from which the real estate cost was 35 per cent and the remaining 263 million roubles was real money.

The history of Russia is rich with its own experience of the establishment and development of all forms of public care. Established traditions are still relevant today, when the demand is especially acute for further maintenance and development of existing state public care structures and the establishment of new forms of care.

As is shown by domestic and foreign experience, the very definition of charity has gone through substantial changes, and the whole basis of charity has changed during the process of social development and industrialisation. Individual mercy was replaced by the social obligation of society.

Family Planning Services in Modern Russia
During the Soviet period, all mother and child protection functions were entrusted to state medical bodies. Social (charity) work was ended as a self-sustaining activity of the medical services. Medical workers themselves were also charged with certain functions of social service. How this work was fulfiled depended largely on the personal attributes and skills of the physicians and nurses.

The family planning theme, as it exists today, is not something new in Russia. The Soviet Union was one of the first countries in the world to begin theoretical research on the practical results of birth-rate control.

In the 1920s and 1930s considerable work was done in liberalising abortion legislation (1920). It was agreed that the next move should be a basically new approach to birth-rate control problems through the proliferation of contraceptives. To this end, as early as 1925 a Commission for Contraceptive Studies was set up within the Mother and Child Department of the USSR People's Commissariat of Health. The Department included a research section and a production laboratory. Massive dissemination of contraceptives was intended through obstetric stations, maternity consultations, mother and child houses, rural medical stations and women's diseases dispensaries.

Because of political pressures, since 1930 all prerequisites for establishing a family planning system in the USSR practically vanished. In 1930 abortions without medical grounds were legally banned and not until 1955 were abortions again legalised. In the 1960s research on the after effects of abortion and new research on prophylactic devices were revived but previous traditions and attitudes had been lost.

Moreover, the basis for formulating state policy concerning the family was the so-called 'interferences' concept. This concept was supported by the following premises: (1) every human being has the primordial need of a big family; (2) the necessity for birth control exists only as long as there are external causes interfering with the satisfaction of this need (that is, living conditions); (3) if these external conditions are changed the birth rate will increase and the number of abortions will go down. State policy was not aimed at family planning but at enhancing people's living standards as quickly as possible.

In the 1970s these theoretical premises were altered in favour of the developmental needs of children, a concept which incorporated medical, psychological, demographic and sociological approaches. The concept was based on a premise that a family itself has to plan the number of its children, depending on its own objectives. Yet society can influence the birth rate indirectly through increasing the populations awareness and through its social policies regarding health. During the 1970s opinions on the social nature of reproductive norms began to take shape. However, numerous publications in the late 1970s and early 1980s contributed practically nothing new to the theory of family planning. Research remained a medical concern and the number of abortions continued to be very high.

An experiment in the 1960s, ordered by the USSR Ministry of Health, explored reducing the number of abortions through wide use of contraceptives. This study identified the low quality of native contraceptives, their low efficiency (under 20 per cent) and inconvenience in their use. The study also noted the negative attitude of some leading medical experts to modern, especially oral, contraceptives. As a result, women did not trust the contraceptives and refused to use them.

Because there was a lack of purposeful social services in this area, the main body of Russia's population have had to content themselves with relatively scant information and there has been little education about contraception. This has been compounded by an insufficient quantity, and low quality and limited variety, of available contraceptives. Especially lacking has been access to oral, hormonal contraceptives since Russia has not had the productive capability for producing these. This has resulted in the fact that even in the 1990s, only 22 per cent of fertile women in Russia are involved in controlled contraception. Yet doubling the number of contraceptive users could reduce the number of abortions by 40 per cent to 50 per cent.

The Russian Family Planning Association (RAFP) points out that Russia's population is robbed of the right to safe sex and contraception while throughout the modern civilised world contraception options and information about methods are available to everybody.

Abortions in Modern Russia

Abortion still remains the main 'method' of family planning in Russia and this problem is extremely acute. Despite the falling birth rate in Russia, the number of abortions has not changed at all. The abortion rate in the Russian Federation remains today one of the highest in the world (about four million a year). On the average every woman living in Russia undergoes four to five abortions during her fertile period. Annually about 190,000 women break off their first pregnancy.

The majority of artificial abortions are done for social reasons. The lack of a systematic approach to solving family planning problems, as well as of providing appropriate medical and social services, makes artificial abortion the main means of birth control. About 30 per cent of maternity deaths are due to abortions. Abortion consequences are truly dramatic in Russia since besides the high maternity death rate abortions are the cause of high infant mortality, premature delivery complications in birth and pregnancies, deteriorated health of children and eventually of the nation as a whole. According to statistics and research findings the health of girls, pregnant women and newly born babies' mothers is adversely affected by previous abortions. During 1985 to 1992, the anaemia rate in pregnant women increased by 4.5 times, the toxicosis rate doubled and the normal birth rate was not more that 45 per cent.

Two years ago an international research panel questioned 375 Russian gynaecologists on the main reasons for such high abortion figures in Russia. The priority rating is the following: (1) sexual ignorance, (2) male partners' indifference and (3) lack of contraceptives. It should be noted that the questionnaires of the International Women's Centre (IWC) 'Woman's Future' project described later in this chapter produced similar results. In both cases the first reasons for abortion were of a social nature and could be dealt with to some extent by increasing education and awareness. The third reason is social in the sense that if economic conditions and trade policies were changed, oral contraception could be made available through imports, or if production facilities were available in Russia to make better quality contraceptives, they would be used more widely.

Non-Governmental Agencies and Family Planning

Even before planned parenthood programmes became realised in modern Russia, non-governmental organisations anxious about the situation began to implement independent programmes. The non-governmental International Women's Centre's 'Woman's Future' project started developing its model programme in 1990 and started providing family planning services in 1992. The project is financed by the International Department (FPIA) of the American Planned

Social Work and Family Planning in Russia: A Public Health Perspective

Parenthood Federation (APPF) for the period 1992-1996. The main task of the project is to educate people about the benefits to be derived from a serious attitude toward birth control and to demonstrate that family planning affects both the individual's and the family's quality of life.

Non-governmental organisations working in this area often have more success making contact with hard-to-reach groups such as young people, national minorities, rural populations and representatives of various confessions and beliefs, than do government agencies.

Phase One of the project recognised that a woman's *total* health should be valued. This premise changes the nature of the client:staff relationship, in that staff seek to make their services readily available and visible, not waiting for women to come to them. The project seeks (1) to attract women's attention to these issues, (2) to help women cope with them, (3) to preserve women's health, and (4) to promote or maintain a supportive atmosphere in the home.

In Phase Two, social and educational services are provided to various sections of the population: factory workers, office workers, students, scientists, teachers, rural communities, representatives of national and religious minorities. The approach takes into account the differing perceptions and behaviours of each group and designs approaches accordingly.

In Phase Three, the programme becomes more complex. It involves training and retraining of medical doctors and assistants, social workers and administrative personnel. Content includes family planning philosophy and issues, technical information, and skills needed for delivering family planning information. Training also provides information materials and a supply of contraceptive devices. All services and materials provided under the programme are free of charge.

In Phase Four, planned parenthood services are set up and are offered on site. This project began in 1992 and is named 'Russia-01: Women's Health Through Birth Control'. The model to be created is oriented toward work with different social groups on the basis of age, ethnicity, region, and occupation. These groupings will determine different approaches to the establishment of the medico-social services provided. Project sites include eighteen Moscow industrial sites, two institutions of higher education, and a small project in Irkutsk for a northern national minority. The main task in this phase is to find personnel and to train them, to organise medical and social services at the sites, to prepare and distribute information materials. Social workers are chosen and trained to provide direct services to clients.

In 1993 the 'Russia:01' project expanded to a rural region. Special training was conducted to improve qualifications of medical specialists, female obstetrician assistants from the obstetrician services (FAPS), social workers and, for the first time in the programme's history, to train volunteers. An educational course about family and sexual problems for teenagers began in one Moscow school, study guides were prepared and two training courses were held for teachers. Students enrolled were able to use the Centre's family planning consultants on a weekly basis.

During 1994 the project continues to expand to new regions. Each regional programme is different, depending on regional needs and characteristics. In one region, a model for mixed village-city services was implemented. In another, planned parenthood services were established in ecologically contaminated areas. The first medical-social planned-parenthood services opened in one of the Muslim republics of Russia.

Analysis of Work to Date

Three years of practical work with staff and clients now permit a summary of some results. The project served up to 21,400 clients. For distribution of clients according to social structure see Table 1.

Table I Social Structure of Clients, 1992–3

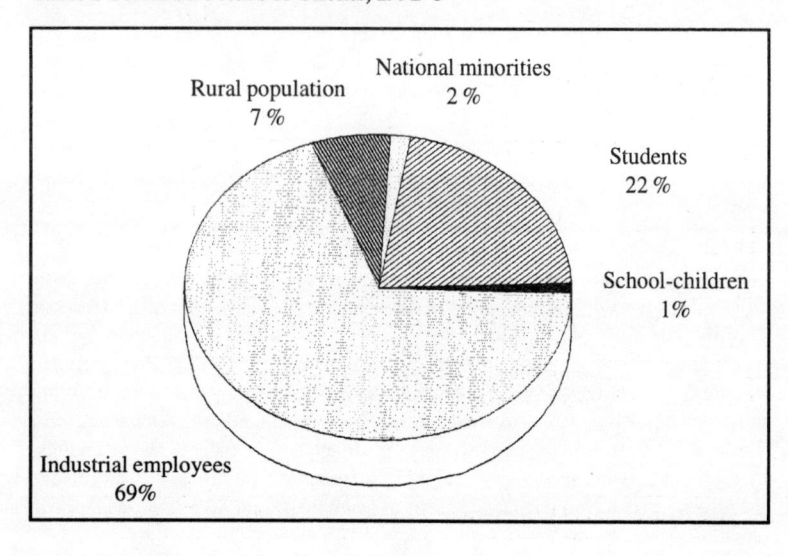

- Rural population 7%
- National minorities 2%
- Students 22%
- School-children 1%
- Industrial employees 69%

Women of fertile age made up 60 per cent - 92 per cent of those served. The rate of their repeated use of family planning service is very high, reaching 93 per cent - 94 per cent in some cases. The pattern and type of contraceptive use have changed, as shown by results in Table 2.

Table 2 Types of Contraceptive Used, 1992-3
percentage of clients using contraceptive

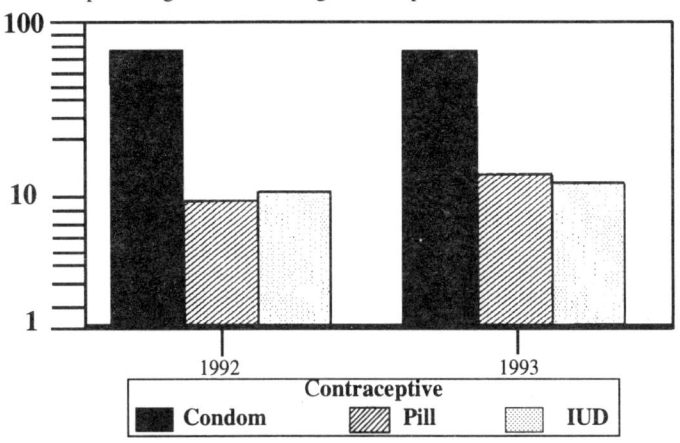

Table 3 Oral Contraceptives Use, 1991–3
percentage of clients using oral contraceptives

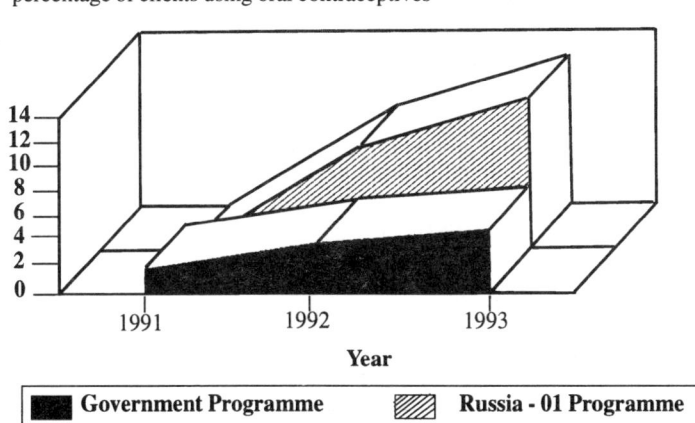

Taking into account that when the programme was initiated only about 10 per cent of future clients used modern contraceptives (such as tablets) it is possible to compare the use of modern contraceptives in Russia generally and among the programme's clients.

Programme participants stated they suffer for lack of 'clear information'. The majority were annoyed that their first experience of communication with a doctor was not helpful. 'He had no time to settle my problems' and 'I had no desire to visit him again' were typical comments. Women's reluctance to ask questions of doctors may be due to fear of creating dependency or of being rejected. It may also be due to the doctor's inability to provide information in a clear and concise manner. Sometimes it may be due to the doctor's inability, because of time pressure or lack of skill or knowledge, to view the woman as a whole person rather than as an object in the gynaecological chair. These factors contribute to mis-information and rumours which lead to women's reliance on folk-tales and remedies, low quality literature and video-tapes, and advice given by casual friends.

Men working at the programme sites were also eligible to use family planning services. At first, men were not willing to enter a typical 'women's' consulting room, but doctors and social workers gradually educated men about the project. Men tend to hold the belief that concerns about family planning and a woman's health are a woman's business. There is now increased understanding that this is also a male responsibility. A number of men requested services for their wives, who were not working on the project site, and staff made a positive decision to meet these requests.

At the end of the analysed period, clients indicated the factors which influenced their use of the programme. They named the following: (1) a wish to have valuable information and (2) to be able to introduce family planning to all family members. This supported the conviction that planned parenthood services should be family focused and create an atmosphere where both men and women can address these issues and request services.

Training of social workers in this project focused on the specific needs and desires of the areas of the population with which they had to work. From 1992 to 1993 60 industrial workers, 122 school-teachers and 30 volunteers from rural regions were trained as social workers according to procedures developed by the International Women's Centre.

Education for Professional Social Work Training

It is in both the medical and the social service spheres that social workers address issues regarding the health care of mothers and children. When analysing potential contributions professionally trained social workers may make to the well-being of women during their childbearing years, it should be noted that in Russia the social service system is just beginning to acquire a new identity. The new profession of social work has just been established and shows promise as an effective way to address the social aspects of many health and medical problems.

Traditionally, relations between the family and the state took place only when the family took the initiative. The role of the new social work profession, however, is not limited to rendering help authorised by the state and sought out by families. Social workers also fulfil a mediating function, seeking to offer to families the state's services. The social worker has no legal right, nor does any social worker wish to claim the right, to interfere with family life, for throughout the civilised world private life is protected from state intervention. Accordingly, the decision to accept or to reject the social worker's assistance in family planning depends on the family's wishes. However, the family's decision also depends on the effectiveness of the social worker and the professional status and importance of this work as evaluated by society.

In Russia today those practising social work must gain official certification. Official status for the profession was granted *pro forma* by the Law on Youth Policy in the USSR in 1991 and by the State Committee for Labour and Social Problems Order on 23 April 1991. This order approved the adding of a position, 'the specialist in social work', to the qualifications register. An additional incentive for more-intensive work on social work theory and practice was the Russian Federation President's Decree in January 1992. He outlined the 'first priority measures for realisation of the World Declaration on securing children's survival, protection and development' in the 1990s and for fostering 'the creation and strengthening of the territorial network of new institutions for social aid to the family and children (centres for family social aid, psychological and pedagogical advisory services, family planning centres, medical and pedagogical schools . . .)'.

At the same time as this concept of social services for the population of the Russian Federation was being created projects of social work with different population categories were also organised. Yet even now social work is not actually recognised as a fully fledged profession. Moreover, there is no final decision on a structure of the state social service. Generally, social service provision follows departmental patterns. The former Minister of Russia's Ministry of Social Protection stated that social work, covering in essence various departments' domains, must be organisationally divided between them, and so it is today. The most developed network of social institutions is established within the Ministry of Social Protection. Other ministries and departments have their own social services.

In the Ministry of Health system, family planning centres and some other programmes serve this purpose. However, the social work mechanisms currently set up in the health care system mean in effect charging practising physicians and the medical system with social work functions. In principle, this is possible. An example of this approach is the pre-birth patronage carried out by a nurse from the children's polyclinic at least twice during the pregnancy period. The purpose is to get acquainted with the child's prospective living conditions and to identify possible domestic and social risks which may affect the child's life. Another example of social functions performed by physicians is a medical care system for babies. This is the work done by district paediatricians.

It must be asked, however, if this transfer of social work tasks to medical workers is effective and cost efficient. Medical workers may make important contributions to the solution of many social ills. However, they cannot and must not assume sole responsibility for solving the complex social problems facing their patients. Doing so may be to the detriment of their proper medical functions.

It is impossible, and inadvisable to try to maintain the *status quo ante*, particularly in light of the country's transition to new economic relationships which will govern the medical care system. In some medical institutes and schools, training programmes are being augmented with more social content; for example, the legal, medico-social and economic aspects of health care. This will undoubtedly help medical personnel to better understand the psycho-social aspects of health care and illness so this is a positive development. Such programmes are already adopted in the medical institutes in Moscow and St Petersburg. A few experiments are under way in Nizhny Novgorod to train social workers for children's polyclinics.

As for the family planning services, in newly set up Family Planning Centres which were formerly mainly established on the basis of women's consultations sites, social work has not yet found its place even though its importance is being declared at all levels. Social work is regarded as having a professional sphere of work in a few regional family planning centres — for instance, in Izhevsk, Samara, Irkutsk and Altai territories. In these centres, the administrations not only understand the necessity of such work but because of their own experience realise its importance.

In recent years the role of social organisations in solving family planning problems became much more prominent. Among them are the Russian

Social Work and Family Planning in Russia: A Public Health Perspective

Association for Family Planning which is doing much to improve information support; the Family and Health International Association, one of the first to tackle reproductive problems; and the Fund for Mother and Child Protection. All of them do new and useful work for mother and child health care.

However, many barriers hamper further development of family planning programmes in Russia. First is the lack of state financing. Although this might be justified on the basis of the difficult economic situation in Russia, this lack of funding results in increasing numbers of women experiencing poor health, increasing numbers of children born with health problems, and large medical expenditures which could be avoided were family planning services available.

Another barrier concerns the availability of high quality contraceptive devices. Contraceptives produced in Russia tend to be of substandard quality. For oral contraceptives, the country is dependent on those imported from other countries.

It must also be ascertained how long the charitable, non-government organisations now providing the bulk of family planning education and service will be able to maintain their programmes. It is questionable whether any amount of charitable giving and any number of non-governmental organisations can maintain the scope of family planning services required in Russia. It is also questionable if the government could effectively perform this function on its own, even in times of less stringent economic problems. A question for the future is what kind of 'partnership' will evolve between the government and non-governmental organisations. Only in such a partnership arrangement will it be possible to provide family planning programmes capable of meeting the needs in Russia. Such partnerships must exist at the central government level as well as the local, regional level. Regional authorities are currently trying to solve health care financing problems with varying success.

There is no doubt, however, about the need for establishing an autonomous social work profession and social service programme which may, as part of their undertaking, make significant contributions to family planning endeavours. Neither medical personnel alone nor other ministries and departments with joint efforts can overcome the ever-growing deficiency of social aid. Therefore the first and foremost task in establishing social services and social work is not only developing theoretical concepts and models but also assuring their practical application.

The value base of the emerging social work profession rests on the premise that, in a humane environment, human beings are not unduly exposed to pain and suffering. This premise should certainly hold true when it comes to serving women of childbearing age and meeting their expressed needs.

References

Betskoy I.I. *General plan of Imperial Foundling Hospital for the brought children and of Hospital for poor mothers in Moscow.* St-Pt., 1889.

Charitable Russia. History of the state, public and private charity in Russia. St-Pet., 1901.

Grebesheva I. An interview in *Family Planning.* 1994 N 1.

Grigorieva N.S., Matveichik Z.Ya., Pelikhova L.S. *Sociological report* by Program 'Russia-01. Woman health through the birth-rate control'. Period 'A', Period 'B' 1993-1994.

Komisova N.A., Lebedinskaya O.I., About the role of social workers in solving medical and social problems. *Col. Social work.* M., 1992, N 1.

Lisitcin, Yu.P., Polunin N.V. *Social medicine and health care management. Training programmes for medical-social disciplines.* M., 1992.

Neiding I.I. *Medical societies of Russia.* Published according to the order of the executive committee of XII International doctors congress. M., 1893.

Panphilova A. On the ways of interchange. Exclusive interview in *Social work* 1994, N 1-4.

Social Work in Health Care Organisation M; Dept. of Family, Women and Child Problems of Russian Ministry of Social Protections VNIK. Scientific, Methodological and Legal Bases of the Activity for Social Work Specialists, *Common to All Mankind Values Centre* Social Work in Health Care Organisation m., 1992.

The interview of deputy Health Care Minister of Russian Federation N.N. Vaganov in *Family Planning,* 1993 N 3.

Vaganov N.N. About the state and the perspectives of social workers service development in the field of maternity and child protection. *Col., Social work, M.,* 1993, N 1.

Veselov N.T. About medical and social patronage in the maternity and child protection system. *Col., Social work.* 1993, N 1.

Veselovskiy B.B. *The Zemstvos history during 40 years.* St.-Pet., 1909-1911 vv.1-4.

Visser A.F. (Belgium), Briniks N. (New Zealand), Remenik L. (Israel) *Family planning in Russia: experience and attitude of Russian gynaecologists. Materials of social interrogatory.* 1992.

Chapter 7
Public Health and Preventive Strategies: Social Work Practice, HIV Disease and AIDS

Gary A. Lloyd

Introduction

Individuals, communities, states and nations throughout the world are confronted with a major public health crisis created by the rapid spread of the Human Immunodeficiency Virus (HIV), the cause of HIV disease, and the individual and social consequences of its end-stage, Acquired Immunodeficiency Syndrome (AIDS). Initially viewed as a slow plague which probably would take at least a generation to unfold, the 'volatile, dynamic and unstable' HIV/AIDS epidemic might now be out of control (McLaughlin, 1988; Mann, Tarantola, and Netter, 1992). HIV disease is everywhere, and does not respect national boundaries. Although many governments chose to deny that HIV could become entrenched in their nations, and thwarted early appeals for prevention campaigns, there is now international mobilisation of public health prevention and counselling services through the World Health Organisation Global Programme on AIDS, national AIDS prevention programmes, and non-governmental organisations. It is now well documented that HIV/AIDS is a pandemic. AIDS cases have been reported officially in 164 countries (Mann, Tarantola and Netter, 1992).

Although low prevalence and incidence of HIV and AIDS in any given country may lead to complacency by government agencies, medical personnel and social workers, the steady progression of the virus, once established, cannot be stopped.

Social workers, with their knowledge of human behaviour and social systems, and their clinical skills focusing on psychosocial issues, represent a professional group with significant contributions to make that will:

- help prevent the spread of HIV and thereby reduce the spread of AIDS;
- provide care and comfort to those afflicted by the virus;
- develop and support the services needed by care givers and families and staff members providing direct care to those with AIDS.

The public health social work role provides a framework for social work intervention in primary prevention programmes — programmes specifically designed to prevent the spread of HIV. The clinical social work role provides the framework for secondary prevention — the early identification and treatment of those at risk and/or early identification and treatment of those affected. The clinical social work role also supports social work involvement with caregivers and families. The community development and resource development role provides the framework for social work advocacy, outreach and development of services necessary to serve this population.

The conception of social work practice in relation to HIV and AIDS rests on both generalist and specialist knowledge and skill. It requires a systems orientation to practice and the ability to intervene at multiple systems levels (individual, family, group, community and social policy).

This chapter presents the basic knowledge about the transmission of HIV disease and AIDS which is essential to social work practice in this problem area. It stresses the public health educational role in primary prevention — a social work role that is primarily concerned with slowing the spread of HIV.

Social workers have a major role to play in developing and implementing primary prevention campaigns. Such campaigns are the main line of defence against HIV transmission in all parts of the world. They are especially critical in countries which as yet do not have the capacity to: (1) screen and test the blood supply; (2) offer widespread HIV antibody testing; (3) provide disposable gloves, syringes and other medical supplies; and (4) develop additional medical facilities to take care of medical case loads steadily increased by HIV infection and AIDS.

HIV Disease: HIV Infection and AIDS

Infection with the Human Immunodeficiency Virus is the beginning of a disease process that is continuous and progressive (Volberding, 1992). The Human Immunodeficiency Virus is a retrovirus which mutates quickly and invades and destroys the human immune system in a way not yet clearly understood. The virus attacks cells, renders usually protective antibodies useless, and replicates within cells. The resulting infection ultimately leads to the fatal condition called Acquired Immunodeficiency Syndrome (AIDS). HIV disease begins with infection with HIV, passes through an asymptomatic period which is highly variable in duration, continues to development of symptoms and opportunistic infections or diseases then culminates in the complete breakdown of the immune system, and death.

There is neither preventive nor prophylactic vaccine to prevent or control HIV infection and there is no cure for AIDS. Infection with HIV is considered to be lifelong, and it is believed that AIDS is invariably fatal. Thus it presents to social

*Public Health and Preventive Strategies: Social Work Practice,
HIV Disease and AIDS*

work practitioners the special psycho-social issues and problems associated with any life-threatening illness plus additional psychosocial issues related to the stigma and myths regarding the illness itself.

HIV probably has infected human beings for more than 20 years, but less than 100 years (Gallo and Montagnier, 1988). AIDS was first identified in the United States in 1981 as a puzzling set of unusual symptoms and rare conditions, such as a form of cancer known as Kaposi's sarcoma. It was affecting homosexual and bisexual men. Subsequently, HIV infection and AIDS were discovered to be spreading rapidly among heterosexual men and women in Africa. Although homosexual men continue to be most at risk of infection in north America and western Europe, heterosexual men and women and their children are being affected in growing numbers. By the turn of the century, AIDS is likely to be a heterosexual disease everywhere in the world (Moss and Bachetti, 1992).

Because of under-reporting or inadequate monitoring systems, it is difficult to assess the actual numbers of HIV infected people in the world. It was estimated at the end of 1993 that there were more than 14 million HIV-infected worldwide. Of those, the World Health Organisation Global Programme on AIDS estimated that 50,000 live in eastern Europe, Russia, the Commonwealth of Independent States and central Asia (WHO/GPA, 1994). These low numbers of reported cases of HIV infection are deceptive and should not be grounds for complacency. Under-reporting, delayed reporting, and misdiagnosis distort the true extent of the pandemic. Once HIV appears in a population, it will spread rapidly and inevitably. Because of the long asymptomatic period, HIV may be present but ignored for a long period of time. By the time symptoms of HIV disease appear, the virus has been silently spreading. Infected people who are unaware of their infection, are infecting others. AIDS is the inevitable outcome of HIV infection. At the end of 1993, the World Health Organisation Global Programme on AIDS estimated that more than three million cases of AIDS in adults and children had occurred worldwide (WHO/GPA, 1994).

Prevention Strategies
Because there is no vaccine or cure for HIV infection or AIDS, the only method of slowing the spread of infection is through prevention programmes. Such programmes succeed best when they are part of a public health strategy at all levels of governance, and are aimed particularly at groups or individuals who are known to be at high risk of infection.

Social workers must be both recipients and providers of accurate information about HIV and AIDS. As recipients of information, their practice can be informed. As providers of information, they can help inform the public and other professionals with information about HIV transmission and the progression from HIV infection to AIDS. Information must be supplied to physicians and health care workers at all levels — particularly in primary care settings — and to social workers, educators and clergy. Specific information about the nature of HIV disease, its modes of transmission and prevention must also be presented to the public through all types of electronic and print media.

Working as members of multidisciplinary teams, social workers designing prevention-oriented primary prevention programmes have found that giving explicit information about transmission and prevention is critically important but often difficult to accomplish. Sex and blood are involved in HIV transmission. In many cultures, open discussion about sex, sexuality, or other intimate topics is viewed negatively. In some cultures, blood itself may have ritualistic or sacred meanings. Prevention of HIV requires openness about sensitive issues usually not talked about in polite society, or in mixed company, so a particular culture or belief system may lead to condemnation or punishment of people who try to give explicit HIV-prevention messages. Devising culturally sensitive, acceptable, and effective prevention messages is a critical task for social workers everywhere in the world. Fostering an environment where critical issues can be discussed openly and rationally is another task facing social workers in all parts of the globe.

Transmission of HIV Infection

Once people become aware of the existence of HIV, it is not uncommon for rumours and fear to spread about how HIV infection might be transmitted. It is often assumed that a person might become infected simply by touching an infected person. Such fears are one source of the stigma attached to people with HIV disease. HIV is *not* transmitted by casual contact nor is it spread through coughing, sneezing, touching, or use of toilets or swimming pools. Mosquitoes or other insects do not serve as vectors for HIV transmission although that is a commonly expressed fear in many parts of the world.

Social workers perform an essential function and alleviate unnecessary distress when they provide accurate information to the public, to families and to individuals affected by the virus regarding the transmission of HIV infection.

HIV infection can be transmitted only in the following ways: (1) unprotected (that is, without use of condom) sexual intercourse (vaginal, anal, oral) when one of the partners is infected with HIV; (2) exposure to infected blood (through blood transfusions or blood contaminated syringes and needles or other instruments) or to infected donated body organs or semen; and (3) passage of infection from mother to foetus or infant before, during or shortly after birth.

Sexual transmission
Heterosexual intercourse is the major mode of transmission globally. Unprotected penetrative vaginal or anal intercourse is the most frequent mode of transmission. The degree of risk of oral sex is not yet established, although probably lower than the other two which are designated as high risk practices. Male-to-female transmission appears to be higher than female-to-male, but the degrees of risk are not definitively known (Osmond, 1990; Padian, Shiboski, and Jewell, 1991). Risk of infection through unprotected sexual intercourse rises proportionately with the number of sexual partners. Although transmission can occur in a single sexual contact, multiple sexual partners increase the likelihood of risk (Peterman, Cates, and Curran, 1988). The already high efficiency of sexual transmission of HIV appears enhanced by the presence of co-factors (that is, another disease or assault on the body), such as sexually transmitted diseases.

Social workers who serve populations likely to have multiple sexual partners may inhibit the spread of HIV by educating clients about this risk factor.

Transmission through blood
Receipt of infected blood or blood products is the most efficient means of HIV transmission. The risk of acquiring infection through transfusion of infected blood is very high, ranging in probability from 90 to 100 per cent (WHO/GPA, 1994; Lifson, 1992). In areas of the world where resources are inadequate to support blood transfusion testing and screening programmes, risk of infection through transmission in medical settings is high. Since 1985, the blood supply used for transfusions in north America, western Europe, and some other parts of the world has been protected through serological screening for HIV, elimination of HIV positive blood donations, and excluding blood donors who are assessed to have been at risk of infection.

Transfusion is not the only means of transmission through blood. Unsterile medical instruments used for injections or drawing blood can be implicated. The blood products used by haemophiliacs can also be sources of transmission in areas of the world where heat-treatment of factor VIII and factor IX is not available.

Social workers serving those with health-related problems may wish to include information about blood transfusions as part of their medical history taking in health care settings or settings serving those with health-related problems.

In north America and western Europe, injected drug use has been a rapidly growing source of transmission. Reports of increasing injected drug use in eastern Europe, Russia and the Commonwealth of Independent States suggest that transmission through shared, contaminated, drug-injecting syringes and needles will also increase there. Syringes and needles used to inject heroin, cocaine or other drugs can become contaminated when even a small amount of blood is drawn into the syringe or needle. During subsequent use of a shared needle, infected blood can be injected into another person, establishing a chain of infection among those using the same equipment. Needle exchange and clean-needle programmes have been successful in western Europe and parts of north America, but are controversial in that many people believe such prevention strategies condone the use of injected drugs. Social workers serving alcoholics and other drug users must therefore include information about HIV transmission in their work with these people.

Mother-to-child transmission

The efficiency of mother to child transmission appears to vary in different parts of the world. One set of data estimates the risk of mother-to-child transmission at 13 to 32 per cent in the industrialised countries and from 25 to 48 per cent in developing countries (Dabis *et al.*, 1993). The risk of transmission depends upon a variety of factors which include the timing of maternal infection in relation to pregnancy, the mother's immunologic and overall health status, presence of sexually transmitted disease, premature delivery, and, possibly, the gestational age of the foetus at the time of maternal infection (CDC, 1987b; Lifson, 1992; Newell and Peckham, 1993, S93; Peckham, 1993). Infection may also occur during delivery through exposure to infected blood.

Pregnancy may act as a co-factor for an infected woman and may increase the risk of accelerating the progression from HIV infection to end-stage disease (AIDS).

A critical aspect of mother-to-child transmission has to do with the risk of breast milk given to their infants by infected mothers. Although data are still somewhat contradictory, it has been assumed that HIV-infected women, irrespective of the timing of their infection, have a 25 per cent likelihood of transmitting HIV through their breast milk (Heymann, 1992).

Counselling about breast feeding is a delicate and uncertain task for social workers. If adequate and clean prepared formula is available, infected mothers should make use of it. If formula is unavailable, prohibitively expensive, or can be mixed only with contaminated water, infected women may need to breast feed their children regardless of the risk.

Again, the necessity of an adequate history and exposure to risk factors is a vital prerequisite if social workers involved with pregnant women are to be able to intervene and prevent unnecessary infection of newborns.

Characteristics of HIV Infection and Disease

The course and consequences of HIV infection are unique in several ways when compared with most other infectious diseases. HIV is a virus which can change itself rapidly, spread from cell to cell, and hide in infected cells without giving its presence away. It attacks and destroys the immune system (Berzofsky, 1991). There is a long asymptomatic period following infection. Consequently, a chain of undetected HIV infection can be created when an asymptomatic, healthy-appearing infected person unknowingly infects others who in turn can unknowingly infect still more.

A virtually universal stigma is attached to HIV infection and AIDS, typically because of cultural beliefs about sexual practices and behaviour. This stigma influences and often slows social responses to the presence of HIV, leading to neglect of individual and family needs for psychosocial services and medical care, and to denial of societal or political support for prevention and care strategies.

The course of HIV disease is unpredictable. Some infected persons live for long periods of time without any indication that their immune system is being undermined. Others begin to show varying degrees of symptoms relatively soon after infection. Symptoms of opportunistic infections or disease may appear episodically or progressively. This erratic pattern creates uncertainty for the infected person and for those who provide care.

This stigma and uncertainty present multiple psychosocial problems for the clinical counselling role of the social worker providing services to those with HIV and the network of services, friends and families relating to them.

Although the pace of the progression from infection to disease is unpredictable, the basic sequence of events is well documented. 'Markers' of progression are included in case definitions of HIV disease developed by the World Health Organisation Global Programme on AIDS and the Centres for Disease Control and Prevention in the United States. In the primary HIV infection period, which begins one to three weeks after infection and continues for another one or two weeks, most persons (estimates range from 50 to 90 per cent) develop malaise, fever and headaches of an influenza-like nature These symptoms are frequently self-limiting and transient and are frequently misdiagnosed if an HIV risk history is not taken into account by attending medical or social work staff.

Within one week to three months of infection, the body produces an antibody response to the invasive HIV. These antibodies are the immune system's mechanisms for responding to and defeating invading bacteria or viruses. In the instance of most infections, antibodies are able to protect the body against foreign elements. With HIV, however, antibodies are inadequate to suppress replication of the virus. This is because HIV causes a loss of crucial helper T cells which leads to deterioration of the immune system (McGrath, 1990; Weber and Weiss, 1988). The time between infection and the appearance of antibodies is known as the 'window period'. Although HIV infection is present in the body, it cannot be detected during this period by the most widely used HIV antibody tests. During this window period, an infected person will produce an HIV negative antibody test but will be capable of transmitting infection to others.

An asymptomatic period of indeterminate length follows the appearance of antibodies in the blood. Although the infected person appears and feels well, the virus continues to replicate itself in the lymph nodes and some other tissues of the immune system (Maddox, 1993). The length of the asymptomatic period varies. Duration may depend upon the source of transmission of HIV and range from ten to eleven years (Volberding, 1992).

Compromise of the immune system continues in the asymptomatic period and culminates in early symptomatic HIV disease. Symptoms may range from minor and mildly uncomfortable to severe and potentially life threatening. Typical symptoms include: diarrhoea; weight loss of ten to fifteen pounds, or 10 per cent of body weight; fever; disease of the lymph nodes; lesions of the mucosal membranes and skin; oral and genital lesions due to herpes virus; and neurological changes.

In the final stage of HIV disease, or AIDS, these and other symptoms and conditions increase in severity. Opportunistic diseases which might be handily defeated by a healthy immune system, such as *Pneumocystis carinii* pneumonia, appear with increasing severity. HIV dementia may also develop along with cancers such as Kaposi's Sarcoma, and viral and fungal infections. Ultimately, HIV destroys the immune system's capacity to defend the body to such a degree that opportunistic diseases and other conditions cannot be overcome, and the infected person dies. Once advanced HIV disease or AIDS is evident, the median survival time in developed countries is nine to thirteen months, but it is much shorter in developing countries.

Because the modes of transmission of HIV infection are attached to sex, sexuality, sexual orientation and drug use, all of which are often culturally proscribed and

Public Health and Preventive Strategies: Social Work Practice, HIV Disease and AIDS

not easily talked about, there is a widespread tendency to view HIV disease in political or moral terms, rather than as the public health issue it is. Moralistic judgements can stand in the way of public health approaches to prevention and care, and can contribute to isolation or withdrawal from or by infected persons and those who care for them.

Most of the new cases of HIV infection in the last decade of the twentieth century will occur in the developing nations. Unlike many chronic diseases which strike the very young or the very old, HIV disease disproportionately affects young people in their most productive and vigorously reproductive years. HIV disease, therefore, is a serious threat to social and economic development, as well as to political stability, because it deprives societies of people who would ordinarily be expected to provide leadership or contribute to the productivity of their countries. Child survival strategies may be completely destroyed by HIV and AIDS.

Multidisciplinary Approaches to Prevention of HIV Transmission

Because HIV and its modes of transmission were established early in the pandemic, social workers, health care professionals, educators and governmental officials knew that prevention of infection was possible, and that organised, collective and collaborative strategies and skills for prevention would be necessary. While such strategies were developed at the international level by the World Health Organisation Global Programme on AIDS and by some national governments, many nations resisted prevention campaigns.

Resistance stemmed from: (1) denial that HIV could make inroads into conservative societies; (2) beliefs that HIV affected only western homosexual men; (3) recognition that primary health care systems were already overwhelmed with other, more visible, and non-stigmatised diseases; and (4) reluctance to promote the kind of explicit public health prevention messages and counselling necessary to alert citizens to the sources of transmission and methods of protection.

Several issues bear upon the success or failure of prevention campaigns which are developed by social workers, health educators and medical personnel. First, information must be given in specific, yet culturally acceptable, terms. This is more easily said than done. In societies where sex and sexuality are not openly discussed, even in same-sex groups, for example, it is very difficult to warn against sexual transmission and to advocate condom use. Yet, if HIV transmission is to be slowed, some culturally acceptable methods must be developed. Second, even when factual information is given in an acceptable format, and is understood by those who receive it, information alone may be insufficient motivation to change the behaviour which places someone at risk of infection. For instance, if a person knows how HIV is transmitted, but continues to have multiple sexual partners, his or her rationale may be that the partners all appear to be healthy and clean. This *perception* of risk is of equal importance with *facts* about risk. Finally, not everyone is able to act upon information which they receive and believe. For example, in many parts of the world women do not have significant personal or social power over their sexual lives. Asking a partner or spouse to use a condom may result in rejection or assault.

The only certain method of preventing sexual transmission of HIV is abstinence. Since this is usually neither personally appealing nor culturally supported, abstinence is not considered by most people to be a viable option. The next line of defence is 'safer sex'. Safer sex involves careful use of condoms from start to finish during vaginal, oral or anal intercourse. The term 'safer sex' indicates that even use of condoms is not 100 per cent safe, because of failure of the condom, or lack of knowledge about proper use. Condom usage has been successfully promoted in many parts of the world. There continues to be resistance, however, on the part of men who claim diminished sexual pleasure, and on the part of some organised religions. Also, condoms are not always available, their quality and storage conditions may be problematic, the cost may be prohibitive, and men may not know how to use them properly.

Where injecting drug use is a significant mode of transmission, prevention efforts focus on providing bleach or other disinfectants to clean needles, or on providing opportunities for drug users to exchange used needles and syringes for new ones.

Preventing transmission from an infected mother to her child involves very complex individual decision making which is usually highly influenced by cultural norms and expectations. Although it might appear that all HIV positive women would avoid pregnancy, this is not the case. Because not every infected mother will give birth to an infected child, a woman may decide to take a risk and become pregnant. Strong cultural pressures on women to bear children, and upon men to father many children, create strong barriers to prevention of mother-to-child transmission. Lack of previous exposure to information about contraception and child spacing may also influence decisions about pregnancy by HIV infected women and their partners.

Social workers and others involved in education and prevention efforts must themselves be comfortable when talking about sex, sexuality, and behaviour which are risky. Giving someone appropriate information about HIV, and

Public Health and Preventive Strategies: Social Work Practice, HIV Disease and AIDS

assessing a person's risk of infection, for example, requires the social worker to take a detailed history of sexual practices and drug use. Unless especially trained to do that, the social worker is apt to talk in such general terms that the necessary specific information is neither obtained nor given. The client may feel threatened or offended and reject the information.

The presence of HIV in the world has required all social workers and health care professionals to talk openly about sex in an unprecedented fashion. Taking a history about risk practices (that is, unprotected sex, injecting drug use) requires skill and self-assurance that is infrequently provided in social work training programmes. In many societies, discussion of contraception and family planning is difficult or discouraged. That difficulty is compounded when prevention of the stigmatised and fatal HIV disease is at issue. Ideally, HIV prevention messages would be freely available throughout the world through posters, leaflets, lectures, and counselling in all primary care facilities and polyclinics as well as through the press, radio and television.

Multidisciplinary Approaches to HIV Antibody Testing and Counselling

A number of laboratory tests are available to detect antibodies to HIV in the blood. Although there are more elaborate and expensive tests which can detect the virus itself, those are rarely used for primary testing. The most commonly used primary tests are varieties of the enzyme-linked immunosorbent assay (ELISA) which detect the retroviral antibodies. Where available, the test is administered twice. If the result is negative, the person at risk is given prevention information and tested again in six months. When the result is positive, another blood sample is tested. If that is also positive, a confirmatory test is given using the more sensitive and expensive Western Blot method.

In many parts of the world, HIV antibody testing laboratories are either not available or not consistently supplied. This fact places an additional burden on social workers attempting to slow the spread of HIV infection. Where testing is available, a critical social work task is to provide pre-test and post-test counselling. Pre-test counselling involves taking a history of sexual or drug injecting practices which may have placed an individual at risk and assessment of how the person might react to a finding of HIV positive status. Post-test counselling includes prevention information for both HIV negative and HIV positive persons.

For an HIV positive person, post-test counselling involves discussion of where to find medical and psychosocial resources; how, when, and whether to tell family, friends and employers; and the emotional and social support which will be needed during the asymptomatic period and the final illness.

Where testing is not available, the basic message must be that every sexual partner or fellow drug injector must be assumed to carry HIV. That is, the social worker emphasises the need for 'safer sex' all the time and for sharing only clean needles. These are very difficult messages for people to take in and act upon consistently. They are often countered by expressions of disbelief or fatalism. All members of the health care team become involved in conveying the appropriate message to the affected individual and/or their partners or family members.

HIV/AIDS, Psychosocial Issues and Social Work Practice
The psychosocial responses to HIV infection mirror the physiological course of infection and disease. People may feel emotionally well and in control for a time, and then move into severe depressive episodes. The many uncertainties about the duration and course of infection induce anxiety, particularly where there is high risk of family and social rejection, where medical facilities are inadequate, and where psychosocial support through individual and family counselling and peer support groups is unavailable. Social workers have major responsibilities for developing and implementing supportive counselling programmes which are culturally acceptable, non-stigmatising, and accessible in hospitals, polyclinics and primary care sites.

A major psychosocial issue for people with HIV infection is that disclosure of the infection itself also discloses behaviour which may have been kept secret (for example, homosexuality, sexual intercourse outside of marriage, drug use). The person must cope not only with the implications of HIV infection, but with fears about maintaining important relationships as well. Because HIV often affects young people, the natural order of life seems reversed, and there is usually considerable fear about death, dying, and leaving behind young children.

People respond to their HIV seropositive status in highly individual ways. Some despair and withdraw. Others vow to fight the virus through medical care, psychosocial support, or alternative medicine. Still others move back and forth between those states. A typical reaction has been described as progression from shock through denial, crisis, transition, fear, depression, panic, guilt, anger, self-pity, bargaining, search for meaning and fighting, to a stage of sense of self, positive action and acceptance (Verlimirovic, 1987). There is usually a sense of multiple losses of health, physical strength, hopes for self and family, and standing in the community. Suicidal ideation is common. Delirium and dementia, which are often seen in HIV disease, may alter a person's impulse control and place him or her at risk of harm to self and others. These manifestations can raise anxiety in family caregivers and in social workers and other health care personnel providing treatment and support if they are not well informed about the course and progression of infection and disease.

Psychosocial manifestations are experienced not only by the infected or diagnosed person but by family, friends, and professional care givers as well. Because of fears about possible social ostracism, family members may be fearful of disclosing the HIV status of the infected person to others, with the consequence that all feel isolated during a time of crisis.

Social Work Responses to HIV/AIDS

Social workers involved in HIV/AIDS prevention and treatment programmes must acquire some basic knowledge, values, and skills (Land, 1992).

Knowledge

- The continuum and progression of HIV disease from point of infection through end-stage disease (AIDS).
- Psychological responses of infected persons and their families.
- Prevention messages which must be given in the context of availability, or lack of availability, of psychosocial supports.
- Working knowledge of treatments available for opportunistic infections and other manifestations of HIV disease.
- Understanding of the dynamics of stigma and discrimination experienced by people with HIV disease, frequently from their families and from professional care givers such as social workers and physicians.

Values

- Respecting individuals who are at risk of infection, infected with HIV, or suffering from end-stage HIV disease, or AIDS.
- Understanding and accepting episodic and sometimes non-compliant behaviour.
- Defining HIV disease as a public health issue, not as evidence of moral failings.
- Viewing and treating the person with HIV disease holistically and as part of a family and social network.

Skill
- Ability to talk comfortably and openly about sensitive topics while, at the same time, respecting cultural norms.
- Confidence in providing social and psychological support to the infected person and care givers.
- Awareness of available primary care and specialised medical treatment facilities, and ability to work within, or to attempt to expand, their policies and procedures in regard to people with HIV disease.
- Ability to identify, clarify, verbalise and analyse in ways which contribute to problem solving related to the many practical and ethical issues and dilemmas which arise in the course of prevention, diagnosis, and treatment of HIV infection and AIDS.
- Forming and conducting support groups for persons affected by HIV disease, including spouses, children, and other family members.
- Developing and implementing culturally appropriate and effective prevention campaigns.
- Informing other social workers and health care personnel about the consequences of stigma on people affected by HIV/AIDS, and about unfounded personal fears of infection through casual contact during the course of treatment.

Conclusion

For all the reasons enumerated in this brief chapter, HIV disease raises many challenges for care givers, and imposes many burdens on people affected by HIV disease. Even when medical and psychosocial resources are readily available, and treatments for opportunistic infections and related conditions are accessible, HIV disease causes severe psychosocial problems for infected persons and family and professional care givers. Those problems are understandably increased in countries and situations where there has been denial that HIV can be present, where cultural prohibitions inhibit prevention campaigns, and where the medical infrastructure cannot sustain adequate or consistent testing and treatment programmes.

Whatever the social environment, social workers serve as: (1) educators of the general public; (2) developers and providers of psychosocial support systems through work with individuals, families and groups; and (3) developers of services which can provide palliative care to those with HIV disease, and (4) developers and providers of preventive information to those who may be at risk.

Public Health and Preventive Strategies: Social Work Practice, HIV Disease and AIDS

HIV and AIDS create enormous challenges for social workers. This incurable infection and disease is present throughout the world. Dealing compassionately with people affected by HIV and AIDS requires social workers to be acutely aware of their own prejudices and biases and to expand their repertoire of knowledge and skills. Similarly, social workers must be prepared to confront and educate the general public and policy makers about the public health crisis created by HIV. HIV disease affects every aspect of public and private life, ranging from the personal consequences for the infected person to the expansion of health care facilities, through creation of social policies related to accessibility of treatment and discrimination.

Because HIV is so pervasive in its impact, social workers must adopt and advocate for holistic and humanistically oriented health and social services for individuals living with HIV and AIDS and the worldwide community of societies which must cope with it.

References

Berzofsky, J. (1991). Approaches and issues in the development of vaccines against HIV, *Journal of Acquired Immune Deficiency Syndrome*, 4, 451-459.

Centres for Disease Control and Prevention (CDC) (1987). Public health service guidelines for counselling and antibody testing to prevent HIV infection and AIDS, *Morbidity and Mortality Weekly Report*, 36, 509-515.

Dabis, F. *et al.* (1993) Estimating the rate of mother-to-child transmission of HIV: Report of a workshop on methodological issues Ghent (Belgium), 17-20 February 1992, *AIDS,* 7, 1139-1148.

Gallo, R. and Montagnier, L. (1988). The AIDS epidemic. In The science of *AIDS: Readings from the Scientific American*, W.H. Freeman, New York, 1-11.

Heymann, J. (1992). Is breast feeding at risk? The challenge of AIDS. In J. Mann, D. Tarantola, and T. Netter (eds) *AIDS in the world: A global report,* Harvard University Press, Cambridge, Massachusetts, 616-629.

Land, H. (1992). (ed) *AIDS: A complete guide to psychosocial intervention*, Family Service America, Milwaukee, Wisconsin.

Lifson, A. (1992). Transmission of the human immunodeficiency virus. In V. DeVita, S. Hellman, and S. Rosenberg (eds) *AIDS: Etiology, diagnosis, treatment and prevention*, 3d ed. Lippincott, Philadelphia, 111-120.

Maddox, J. (1993). Where the AIDS virus hides away. *Nature*, 362, 287.

Mann, J., Tarantola, D., and Netter, T. (1992). (eds) *AIDS in the world: A global report*, Harvard University Press, Cambridge, Massachusetts.

McGrath, M. (1990). HIV: Overview and general description. In J. Cohen, M. Sande, and P. Volberding (eds), *The AIDS knowledge base.* The Medical Publishing Group, Waltham, Massachusetts, 1-3. 3.1.1.

McLaughlin, L. (1988). AIDS: An overview, *New England Journal of Public Policy*, 4, 15-35.

Moss, A. and Bachetti, P. (1992). Editorial review: Natural history of HIV infection, *AIDS*, 3, 55-61.

Newell, M.L. and Peckham, C. (1993). Risk factors for vertical transmission of HIV-1 and early markers of HIV-1 infection in children, *AIDS 92/93*, S91-S98.

Osmond, D. (1990). Sexual transmission of HIV infection: overview. In P. Cohen, M. Sande, and P. Volberding (eds) *The AIDS knowledge base*, The Medical Publishing Group, Waltham, Massachusetts, 1-4, 1.2.2.

Padian, N., Shiboski, S. and Jewell, N. (1991). Female-to-male transmission of Human Immunodeficiency Virus, *Journal of the American Medical Association*, 266, 1664-1667.

Peckham, C. (1993). Report to the IX International Conference on AIDS, Berlin.

Peterman, T., Cates, W., and Curran, J. (1988). The challenge of human immunodeficiency virus (HIV) and acquired immunodeficiency syndrome in women and children, *Fertility and Sterility*, 4, 571-581.

Verlimirovic, B. (1987). AIDS as a social phenomenon. *Social Science and Medicine*, 25, 6.

Volberding, P. (1992). Clinical spectrum of HIV disease. In V. DeVita, S. Hellman, and S. Rosenberg (eds) *AIDS etiology, diagnosis, treatment and prevention*. 3d. ed. Lippincott, Philadelphia, 123-140.

Weber, J. and Weiss, R. (1988). HIV infection: The cellular picture. *The Science of AIDS: Readings from the Scientific American*. W. H. Freeman, New York, 64-73.

World Health Organisation. Global Programme on AIDS (WHO/GPA) (1994). *Global AIDS news*, 1, 11-12.

World Health Organisation. Global Programme on AIDS. *Guidelines for counselling people about human immunodeficiency virus (HIV)*, WHO, Geneva.

Introduction to Strategies for Improving Access, Utilisation and Quality of Service: Two Exemplars

The next two chapters present exemplars illustrating strategies which social workers have adopted in their search for interventions and methods to improve the health status of various populations.

These chapters trace historical developments which involved both proactive and reactive responses from the social work profession. Chapter 8 illustrates the use of multidisciplinary teams in facilitating the move from an institutional base for serving those with mentally handicapping conditions to providing services for them in the community in the hope of promoting a more humanising and humane way of life. This trend away from institutional care has been motivated in many countries by both economic considerations and humane treatment philosophies. For 20 years this trend in the West has given rise to many challenges, opportunities and ethical considerations.

Chapter 8 outlines the demands and challenges faced by social workers trying to establish community mental health services dependent on teams of professionals learning to work together on behalf of individual clients. It draws on experience in Slovenia to explore team building and collaborative practice strategies as a means for improving the quality and outcomes of community mental health services. Working in teams composed of medical and social service disciplines has been viewed as a characteristic of social work practice in health care since the beginning of the profession's involvement in health matters. However, the modern deinstitutionalisation movement, which focuses on prevention of hospitalisation and provision of care in the community, makes new demands on all health care professionals. Special group work, group leadership, process-oriented and advocacy skills are the core elements needed if a multidisciplinary team approach is to be effective.

Chapter 9 examines the need for social work strategies to improve access, quality and outcomes of professional social work services provided to refugees in Hungary. Services are being provided by a non-governmental agency as the country tries to meet the needs of an increasingly heterogeneous population of refugees and immigrants.

It has been estimated that as of March 1994 there were eighteen million refugees on the move in the world but estimates are that there are more than 24 million others that are internally displaced within their own countries. Trapped within their own borders they are exposed to crisis conditions and unable to go anywhere in search of a better life. By the year 2000 it is estimated that 200 – 500 million people will be at least temporarily displaced.

To effectively serve these populations social workers must not only have crisis intervention skills but also an ethnically sensitive model of practice. This means a practice model based on an understanding of cultural pluralism and one that respects differences in world views.

The problem-solving process required to work professionally and effectively with the health and social problems of refugees is highlighted in this chapter. The systems problems inherent in providing ethnic-sensitive practice to people in this type of crisis situation are explored. Left without resources and social supports this population may permanently exhibit the phenomenon of learnt helplessness and may remain despondent and dependent the rest of their lives. Refugees, immigrants and migrants of all races and countries are especially vulnerable to psychosocial stress. Rates of psychiatric hospitalisation and illness events among these groups are ordinarily higher than those of other populations both because of stress factors which influence the immune system and of deteriorated health status due to poor housing, poor nutrition and overcrowding. Rates of psychiatric hospitalisation and illness increase as people face unfamiliar conditions, cultural differences, less social support and more conflict as they try to establish some control over their everyday lives and their future.

A variety of problems present themselves when trying to establish a systems approach to serving this population: these include the degree of latitude governments allow those trying to serve these populations; the fact that these populations represent involuntary groups of clients; and that control of these populations is perceived to be essential by those countries receiving them.

The situation of the internally uprooted threatens to become one of the most explosive issues of the coming decades. Few nations will be exempt and social workers in all countries will be increasingly involved in these developments.

It has been noted that while the past affects and gives shape to problems manifested in the future, social work's major obligation is to attend to current issues. This is true whether it is tending to the needs of those with severe mental distress in their own community or those who are displaced and without community. Understanding another's cultural past, whether in terms of the culture of institutional life or culture of an ethnic group, is especially important for social workers in health care. It is cultural factors which influence health and illness behaviour and the utilisation of health and social services.

Both chapters identify bio-psychosocial factors which influence the social work role and function. Both chapters address problems which must be confronted far beyond the boundaries of Hungary and Slovenia. Social workers in all parts of the world will be addressing the issues raised in chapter 8 and chapter 9.

References

Ely, P. and Denney, D. (1987-1989) *Social Work in a Multi Racial Society*; Gower, Aldershot, England.

Green. James W. (1982) *Cultural Awareness in the Human Services*; Prentice Hall, Englewood Cliffs, NJ, USA.

Helman, Cecil G. (1990) *Culture, Health and Illness* (2nd edition); Wright, London.

Kumabe, K.; Nishida, C.; Hepworth, D. (1985) *Bridging Ethnocultural Diversity in Social Work and Health*; University of Hawaii School of Social Work, Honolulu.

Spector, Rachel. (1985) *Cultural Diversity in Health and Illness*; (2nd ed.); Appleton-Century Crofts, East Norwalk Con. USA.

Wright, Robin. *Los Angeles Times World Report;* 8 March, 1994.

Chapter 8
Teams as Means of Interdisciplinary Collaboration: Developing Community Mental Health in Slovenia

Vito Flaker

Community Mental Health as an Interdisciplinary Arena

Mental distress as a human condition is beyond doubt a complex phenomenon. Being 'mentally ill', 'crazy', 'off the hook', having a 'nervous breakdown' or feeling 'just a little bit down' raises many questions. On one level these are questions about realities of human existence and the construction of human experience. On another level are questions about how the brain functions and its relationship to the entire body. On yet another are questions about a person's role and status, the stigma attached to this condition, questions about the family's and the environments response, and about investments in one's own illness. There are questions of a legal nature regarding responsibility and coercion. Most importantly there are questions about how to treat these conditions: how to help, care and/or cure; and what types of support to offer? Many sciences, disciplines and professions — medicine and psychiatry, psychology and psychoanalysis; philosophy and theology; sociology and anthropology; history and politics; social work and nursing; occupational therapy and art — all deal with mental distress.

Throughout history and across cultures there have been different approaches to this phenomenon. They range from outright coercive approaches using chains and sticks, to trying to accommodate, comfort and persuade. Whatever the approach, there were always many participants involved. Sometimes it was family, sometimes the public or tribe. Frequently it was the healers or the clergy and sometimes a friend. Sometimes madmen were left on their own to be as they were or to wander in a no man's land. But it is only since the beginning of the nineteenth century that the 'lunatics' have been put in asylums. This development came in light of the need for regimentation of society in the wake of the Industrial Revolution.

The medical profession has offered the explanation (or the rationalisation) for this act of asylum and has been delegated the power to control the lives of those who have severe mental illness. This dominance of psychiatry and the 'lunatic asylum' as a symbol for treatment of mentally distressed people lasted for more than a hundred years. There were always other disciplines involved, especially in the twentieth century, as auxiliaries to psychiatry. Recent recognition of how harmful and ineffective incarceration in mental hospitals can be, and the subsequent development of community mental health (CMH), signalled the beginning of interdisciplinarity in dealing with issues connected to mental distress.

There were multidisciplinary teams active within psychiatric institutions, especially the branch that is called social psychiatry, but they operated within the logic of institutions and under the jurisdiction of psychiatrists. Members of the team — psychologists, nurses, social workers, occupational therapists and others — were all congregated together with the patients under the same roof and under the single authority of a hospital superintendent.

Contemporary community mental health (CMH) teams are composed of similar professions, but the pattern of relationships in these teams has changed from a hierarchical to a more egalitarian one. Teams in the community are led by various professionals: nurses, social workers, psychologists and others. Social work, or rather social welfare, has become an important factor since, once it became treated in the community, mental distress ceased to be defined solely as a health problem.

There has also been a change in the view people have about the nature of mental illness or distress. The dominant medical model that portrayed mental distress as an illness that pertained to an individual and had to be diagnosed and cured outside of its social context, has been replaced by a more pluralistic model that contains sociological, anthropological and psychological systems and ecological perspectives. The current tendency is to treat issues of mental health holistically, beginning with the perspective and experience of the user, connected to his or her context and environment. There are still antagonisms, for example, between psychiatrists and social workers, resulting from different theoretical models (medical and social ones). These differences sometimes seen unsurmountable in principle and theory, but practice seems to impose the imperative of joint action and collaboration. Since the user is an entity, he or she cannot be split into parts by professions! If the professions are really committed to the users' good, they have to find the way to put their conceptual differences aside. If this cannot be done, then new models of care and treatment are just bids to acquire more power and develop a new type of colonialisation, this time in the community.

There have been two other recent developments. First is the diffusion of services and, second, the users' movements. The first is a logical development of community mental health. 'Intermediary structures' like group homes, day centres and sheltered workshops are definitely a move away from the 'hard' technology of the asylum towards 'softer' ones of community care. However, these intermediary structures do not lose all the repressive and dehumanising features

Teams as Means of Interdisciplinary Collaboration: Developing Community Mental Health in Slovenia

of the asylums. Although closer to ordinary life of the community, users of services were still 'congregated' users. Partly in response to this and partly, in a strange conjunction with neo-liberal ideology wanting to introduce market-like logic into service provision, a whole array of different forms of individualised service provision has emerged. Under different and awkward names, such as case or care management, care planning, individual service plans, and brokerage, these forms of provision provide individualised planning and funding of services. These result in co-ordination of the services around the needs of a single user and give the user more power to control what is being done to and with him or her.

The second development is the emergence of a new participant in the milieu of mental health. In the 1960s and 1970s the main agents of change were professionals, but in the 1990s the users themselves are active agents for change. Be it fashioned in the style of consumer involvement or the civil liberties movement, self-help, or mere protest of being abused, the voice and impact of users are being felt by campaigns against injustice (Brandon 1991). The user as a person involved in the planning and delivering of services should have an impact on the very nature of interdisciplinarity and add something that might be tentatively named 'transdisciplinarity.'

Interdisciplinary Community Mental Health Work in Slovenia: Description of Project Demonstration and Training

In Slovenia, hospital psychiatry has followed western developments except that there has been virtually no development of community mental health work. Unlike most of the socialist regimes, social work was a known discipline in Yugoslavia but social workers had little skills in community mental health work. There were no voluntary non-government organisations until 1991 although there was a small movement emerging in the late 1980s. In 1991, in a sort of historic compromise with official psychiatry practice and with support of Trieste psychiatric services, a programme called 'Community Mental Health Studies – Training for Psychosocial Services' was started. It was funded by the EEC through the TEMPUS programme. The Triestian psychiatric services have been the primary movers of Italian psychiatric reform (Basaglia 1981, 1987, Ramon and Giannichedda 1988).

The aim of the project was to educate the first generation of Slovenian specialists in the field of community mental health and to create awareness of this issue in the professional and general public. The project was created at a time of rapid change, in an atmosphere when everything seemed possible. The project was co-ordinated by the School for Social Work, University of Ljubljana, with partners in

Italy (Trieste), England and Austria, and with a marginal involvement of a French and a German institution. Both academic and service organisations were involved in the project.

The group of 26 project students consisted of a range of professionals (twelve social workers, five psychologists, four educational workers, three sociologists, two doctors (a psychiatrist and a general practitioner) and a nurse. Most were already working in this or a related field. They were taught by an inner team comprising a co-ordinator and four tutors, who together with the students, underwent the learning experience provided by the teachers from Slovenia and abroad.

The teaching was made up of theoretical presentations, practical workshops and practice placements. Important topics were deinstitutionalisation, action and qualitative research, normalisation, care planning and brokerage. An important feature of the course was to consistently employ feminist and anthropological perspectives. Throughout the course the issue was user involvement and advocacy. Practical workshops were devoted to developing skills like counselling, risk analysis, teamwork, work with networks, and supervision. There was also content on the organisational features of management, fund raising, and work with voluntary organisations. An important feature of the course was a six months' practice period. Half of the students went to Trieste, half to England and one to Austria.

There were a number of lectures for other audiences and numerous consultations to different professionals. In this way information was disseminated among professionals working in the spheres of mental health, general medicine, and social services. There were articles and interviews published in the press, appearances on television and radio. Literature was published in Slovene: manuals, a book, and special issues of the Slovenia Journal of Social Work.

There have been two main outcomes of this project, apart from the knowledge gained and used in the projects that our students set up in the emerging voluntary sector: (1) the emergence of social work as a factor in community mental health and (2) the beginning of the users movement. Although the project was not wholeheartedly accepted by traditional psychiatrists, and changes are not dramatic, there are numerous positive responses. There is now an awareness in Slovene society of the need for deinstitutionalisation and the introduction of community care.

This project was thoroughly interdisciplinary in terms of subjects taught, in terms of students and lecturers and in terms of the public. The merit of this enterprise is that our students learnt to think in interdisciplinary ways in the process of studying together, and they learnt about other disciplines not only from their lecturers and trainers but also from their fellow students.

Teams as Means of Interdisciplinary Collaboration: Developing Community Mental Health in Slovenia

Teams as a Concrete Form of Interdisciplinary Action

Interdisciplinary co-operation is possible on many levels and takes many forms. It happens in education, as in our project; in research when students from different disciplines come together to share different aspects of a single problem; in consultation, when professionals are summoned to help with a particular aspect of a problem that a practitioner, a team or an organisation is facing but does not feel equipped to deal with. Teams are definitely a concrete and widespread form of interdisciplinary action. They require people to come together and to try to do things together, harnessed by the action of achieving a common goal. Incidentally, the original meaning of the word 'team' is 'two or more draught animals harnessed together'!

Payne (1982) defines a collaborative team as having 'common goals and its members, while retaining personal and individual responsibilities, divide up their work so as to make the best of their activities and ensure that they achieve their goals'.

Multidisciplinary teams could be defined as 'a small group of people, usually from different professions and agencies, who relate to each other to contribute to the common goal of meeting health and social needs of one client or those of a client population in the community' (Øvretveit 1993).

It is often said that a group is more than the sum of its parts. But from our everyday experience we all know that working in groups can be frustrating and even detrimental to the goals and tasks assumed. In the area of social work and mental health the traditional method is one-to-one casework, so why would we like to do our work collectively?

There are basically two answers. One is that, because users' needs are complex, teams can best address the complexity. Users of mental health services often present difficult life situations which cannot be dealt with by a single professional, especially given the growing specialisation in the human services. For example, a client needing long term and continuing care will need not only administration of medication but also support with housing, employment, counselling, and easing relationships with relatives and neighbours. These services can be provided effectively only through co-ordination between the participants involved. In this way, the user benefits 'from [a] wide variety of knowledge and method, which cannot be exercised by one practitioner or profession' although 'certain skills and knowledge are common to helping professions' (Falck quoted in Carlton 1984), which in turn makes the integration of the teamwork possible.

Secondly, teams are advantageous for professionals. Professionals need teams for the purposes of dividing work and distributing power. A user's time is finite, so practitioners have to decide how to use it. One could easily imagine that after multidisciplinary assessment of a single user by a team of different professionals, the time needed for implementing all the different treatments could possibly exceed 24 hours a day. The user is more and more divided by the hours of being recipient of different services. So teamwork is an opportunity for the professionals to confront the fact that user's time is finite and to make use of it via establishing their priorities and co-ordination of their activities.

Another raison d'être of teamwork for the professionals is power relations between the professions. Different professions enter teams with different degrees of power in terms of legal competencies, status, and training. Teamwork may be seen either as a melting pot of different powers or as an area of power struggle. For example, a typical hospital-based team can be used as a means of colonising other professions by a dominant medical profession, while in a community mental health team usurpation of power by the newer caring professions can be observed (Hughman 1991). In many cases it is the client who is left the most powerless.

Formal Teams and Informal Networks

Professionals can associate in many different ways. Most professionals collaborate with other professionals informally through more or less regular contacts, seeking advice, consultation or sometimes intervention, when they (or their organisation) are not in a position to provide a required service. On the other hand, there are groups of people who come together (or in some instances are put together) to accomplish some common goal or task. This distinguishes mere work groups from developed collaborative teams (Payne 1982). People who come together do not automatically become a team. A process is needed for a group to learn to function as a team. Payne adds two other styles of teams, which fall somewhere in between: leader-centred teams and individual-centred teams. There are more taxonomies of groups possible , for example according to power structure and group mentality, but their use for any pragmatic practitioner is not much more than to orientate the practitioner to a particular situation.

Most teams are formed around the task at hand. Although it is possible to point out some advantages of team collaboration and collaborative teams, 'ideal types' should not be taken as some normative measure against which *all* teams should be measured. Some types of teams are good in some situations and some in others. In the following passage we shall outline a third type of team.

Teams as Means of Interdisciplinary Collaboration: Developing Community Mental Health in Slovenia

Network-Association Teams, Permanent Teams and Client Teams
Most loose formations are networks of people who know each other, who vaguely have common ideas and values, but who do not necessarily work in the same establishment or profession. For instance, in Slovenia there was a pronounced interest in group work and humanistic psychotherapies in the early 1980s. Although it was headed by some psychologists, there were people from other professions involved — social workers, psychiatrists, occupational therapists, nurses and others. There were some communal events like monthly meetings and summer schools. There were also many informal contacts between the members of this network. The main activity of the network was furthering group work in terms of theory, practical skills and group work techniques and at the same time creating a set of values. Also there was practical help shared between the members in consultation, supervision and some cross-referring of clients.

A similar process was observed in the activities that accompanied and followed our community mental health course. Students met monthly to share their experiences and discuss common issues. In addition, the students met outside this framework, participated in each other's projects, offered views of each other's work and occasionally helped with a colleague's work.

On the other side of the continuum there are formal teams, with designated roles and tasks and established rules of communication and functioning. Sometimes they involve people working in the same establishment and at others they cut across different organisations.

As an example, in conjunction with our educational project there was a group home formed for four men who had been in an institution for many years. This group home was a bit overstaffed because it was the first such project. There were four members of staff: two social workers, one social pedagogue and a general practitioner interested in the development of community mental health. The main organisational principle was that in addition to having their individual duties, each member of staff was a key worker to one of the residents. One of the social workers was the manager, the doctor was in charge of medical matters and liaison to the institution where the residents originated, the second social worker was in charge of maintenance and the social pedagogue was in charge of occupational and leisure activities. This core team was complemented by a psychiatrist and some volunteers. The psychiatrist consulted on psychiatric matters and monitored medications. Volunteers had the role of companion to the residents on their outings and in domestic life as well. The supervision of the team was provided by an international volunteer who had previously been a group home manager in the USA, and later by the management of the voluntary association that established the group home.

The organisation of the team followed two directions. One was the residents, the other the specific areas of different professions and their roles. The first dimension provides residents with a person that they can refer to, that can advocate their interest in the collective situation and see that individual needs and desires of a resident do not get forgotten in the process of teamwork (Brandon 1991). The other dimension allows different professions and individuals to contribute their specific expertise or to develop specific roles that are needed in the team. Developments such as this provide an opportunity to observe a rudimentary form of what can be a 'client team'.

After time spent in the group home convalescing from the debilitating effects of the asylum, one resident began to reown his capacities. Unfortunately this meant that there were difficulties. The group home situation became unbearable for other residents and some staff. After several disruptive incidents, the decision was made that the resident be moved to another location and live on his own. A special budget for this resident and a new staffing arrangement had to be made. His key worker 'moved' with him. Since more support and surveillance than the key worker could provide were needed, the key worker was supported by the group managers and more volunteers were recruited. They formed a special team that was concerned only with this resident's day to day matters. A psychiatrist still remained in charge of monitoring the medication and another psychiatrist, known to the resident from before and having a good rapport, provided counselling services. Together with the social worker of the local social services and the chairman of the association they have formed a wider team that come together (with the client) periodically to review the process and discuss the issues connected with the life of this individual resident.

While client teams are usually connected with the development of a care management system and/or a care management plan, it was not so in this instance. There was a notion of individualised planning involved, but more or less this was an *ad hoc* solution to the problem of managing a group home. Still, this approach identifies a basic feature of this type of team — the professionals come together only for this particular user and the team involves both formal and informal carers. In fact one of the professionals exclaimed in a moment of despair when the resident was 'misbehaving': 'All these distinguished people are coming here because of you and look what you are doing!' And in a way he was right: the user is the king!

The Dynamics of Teamwork
Like other groups, teams go though a developmental process which can be viewed as a series of stages. There are many theories about these stages, which

Teams as Means of Interdisciplinary Collaboration: Developing Community Mental Health in Slovenia

could be described in the following manner (Bion 1963, de Board 1978, Southgate and Randall 1980): (1) there is an orientation phase, when group members want to know what is going on, what is expected of them, and worried about how they are perceived; (2) in the second stage there is more question about purpose; this is also the time for conflicts, when the group really gets going, when conflicts are resolved creatively and the group achieves something; (3) this is followed by relaxation, subsuming the activity, giving finishing touches and closing down. Such an ideal sequence of stages is achieved in favourable conditions and when people take notice of emotional, productive and organisational aspects of working together. Sometimes groups get 'stuck' and become preoccupied with a single aspect of their functioning. Knowledge of group processes, theoretical and experiential, is required for people working in teams and providing group leadership.

Roles in Teams An important part of the dynamics of teamwork has to do with the process that team members experience. Some authors speak of a process in stages of: (1) *role separation* - sticking to the traditional roles and strict role boundaries, (2) *overestimation* of teamwork, (3) *disappointment* (which can cause the introduction of more-rigid schemes), (4) *realistic appraisal* of work done, (5) *accommodation* of differences and complementarily (6) *integration* of role in the team.

Different professionals learn from each other and there is some interchanging of the tasks different people undertake, so there is some overlapping between members' tasks and the blurring of professional roles. While overlapping can be considered an essential prerequisite for teamwork, since there has to be some common ground in order for teamwork to take place, role blurring is a somewhat more difficult concept and opinions on this issue are divided. Some authors (Germain, Carol Bailey1984) say that it leads to 'ambiguity and confusion for patients and families', or unclear roles for professionals. It can also be seen as an avoidance of conflict between some professionals (Carlton 1984) or even lead to deskilling and dissatisfaction with the work.

Others see the process of role blurring as a possibility for creative change. In this view some role blurring is necessary in order that people can grow into new roles which will be specific to a particular team. The idea is that in the process of team development, people will take on tasks which will gradually combine into a role that would be necessary and organically needed in this particular team. Here we have two notions of teams. One corresponds to the idea of a 'melting pot' and another to the 'arena of professional division of work'. To be practical it seems that role blurring is an appropriate process for teams where a team is moving from a very structured and hierarchical organisational basis to a more flexible and egalitarian one and when new skills and roles are needed. An example of this might be transition from a hospital-based team to one that is community based. A certain degree of role blurring is bound to occur in teams where a key-worker system is operating.

Dynamics of Power One can rightly assume that teams are also a means of getting people to do things, making them comply with the goals of a certain organisation. Coming to a group or facing a team certainly means giving up some individual sovereignty. On the other hand teams can also be perceived as an empowering device. Different professionals come to a team with different formal competencies, professional prestige, organisational and institutional prerogatives, and personal force. Much depends on how these will be used in the team. For instance, a psychiatrist who has formal power, like compulsory admission, can decide about this regardless of what the rest of the team think about it. He can consult with the rest of the team members and then reach a decision, or he can delegate his power to the team and work with the team to reach a decision that will satisfy everybody. Note that not only are the rest of the team gaining more power but also the psychiatrist himself. Should he argue about the decision which was made collectively outside the team, his arguments will be sounder and also stronger, since there would be a whole group behind it.

Becoming a Subject Group — A Case for Users' Involvement The real issue of power(lessness) is tied to the issue of users' involvement. Most of the work groups and teams are what Guattari (1972, 1984) terms dependent groups, depending on the hierarchies of the organisations they belong to and the definitions of their goals. Many teams became bound by internal struggles over division of labour and power. This has a mortifying effect on their imagination and creativity. On the other hand there are what Guattari terms subject groups, with their imagery unbounded by dependency ties to hierarchies and exposed to the raw existential matters of death and 'othernesses'.

In the community mental health movement, the existence of subject groups is often related to the user's involvement. The logic is quite simple. If the thing that matters most in providing the services to people in mental distress is their own need, who will be more concerned about fulfiling these needs than the users themselves? In Ljubljana we have had experience with two teams that were led by users and involved various professionals. One was an advocacy project and the other involved an association of drug users. In both instances, leading the project was more than a job for the leader-user. It was a vocation, a concern not only for individual well-being but also for the well-being of the group.

There were two distinctive features in these two teams. First, the distinction between 'them' (users) and 'us' (professionals) that is present in most services and

Teams as Means of Interdisciplinary Collaboration: Developing Community Mental Health in Slovenia

teams somehow disappeared. And second, the language has been transformed from professional jargon to more common language intelligible to everybody. Language becomes critical when users who participate in client teams are not educated or trained in some professional tradition.

What is there for professionals to do if the users are so good and so crucial in running their own services? Although user-run services are a trend, there are two things that professionals can still contribute: power and art. Power is something that is constituent to the professional, without it he or she would not be one. The trick is that the power delegated to the professional can be delegated further to the users. Users can use professional power in several ways: (1) in making their voice heard; (2) in being represented in the formal power structures where professionals already have their niche; (3) in linking with available resources. Skills, thoughts and knowledge can also be shared.

However, strengths of the users may also be their deficiencies. For example, the leader of the drug users project was without proper support from management and had personal problems that led to burn out. He slid back to his drug addiction and finally opted out, leaving his peers sadly disillusioned. The art of the professional would be to be supportive enough without being too patronising and colonising. A difficult art to master given the history of caring and curing professions.

Social Work's Role and Contributions in Interdisciplinary Collaboration
Social work has a special advantage over other disciplines in that it is interdisciplinary in its construction. In professional education, social workers learn principles of almost all that deals with social and human existence and usually continue to use these heterogeneous concepts in their practice. What is even more important is that social workers are unique among practical professions dealing with human existence in that they do not have a temple to their science (Jordan 1984, 1987). Doctors have clinics, teachers have schools, lawyers have courts. These spaces transform everyday ordinary living into specially codified sets of events of health and illness, knowledge and discipline, right and wrong, understood in a special language of the clergy of that special temple. This somehow leaves social workers in ordinary man's land, speaking his or her own language and talking about mundane problems of existence (like what to do with a sick relative, how to get transportation to attend the clinic, where to get money to pay the electricity). In a way social work deals with the problems similar to those of a housewife, figuring out how to make ends meet, although we must say, in more difficult times (unemployment or long-term handicaps, for example) and extraordinary conditions (nervous or financial breakdown, or delinquent act). Another distinctive feature of

social work as a discipline is that it is about *doing* not about *explaining*, as in psychology and sociology. It differs from other practical sciences (medicine, pedagogy, law) in that it does not have preconceived outcomes (standardised cure, education or justice) but just a calculus of improved welfare for singular situations.

So social work in an interdisciplinary setting can:

- translate (using common and ordinary language) between disciplines and professions and between professionals and users and carers;
- link the team processes to the everyday social context of the user and to the institutional realities regarding resources and situations;
- translate theory into action using the immediate potential and avoiding preconceived standardised outcomes.

Tilbury (1993) writes that the contribution of a social worker to mental health teams is to see that the 'sufferer' stays alive: (1) by delicately using power to minimise the risks involved; (2) by providing supervision; (3) by involving networks and preserving and improving quality of life; (4) by specifically contributing to assessment and treatment.

A social worker can contribute to social history and social assessment, highlighting the background of what has been termed mental ill health, that goes beyond the crisis which is to be dealt with. Social work contributes to understanding the personal, social and material context where the distress arose and to understanding the problem as a whole. This will enable the team to link its strategy to the existing potentials in the everyday environment. In many stages of treatment, the social worker's contributions might be team co-ordination, assuming some kind of secretarial role, or providing the information flow that ensures that people know what they are doing.

It could also mean interpreting professional reasoning to users and carers as well as insuring that their voices are heard correctly by the rest of the team. It is of vital importance that the users and carers are not given solutions by the professional team, but that they are presented with the problems that they are to solve. In this way users are involved in the working of the team and in providing for their own well-being (Freire 1972, Rose and Black 1985). This sometimes means involving users, initiating advocacy, and linking to welfare resources which may include informal help or local resources. Social worker's contributions also include seeing that services in the immediate environment, such as a hospital, are integrated into planning, monitoring developments, reporting back and making sure that the team reviews its work periodically.

Teams as Means of Interdisciplinary Collaboration: Developing Community Mental Health in Slovenia

Conclusion

This chapter presented an idealisation of teamwork which to social work practitioners seems distant from the everyday life of social work practice. These are also foreign conceptualisations and it is sometimes difficult to implement concepts that grow in a different social structure and culture. Concepts like professional, self-help, supervision, user, and team may have meanings that are different in Slovenia from the culture in which they originated.

Another problem faced when presented with 'ideal' forms, such as that of community-based services, is that those who are involved in establishing them find themselves in a situation where time runs out. There is so much to do and so little time to do it!

Another frustration stems from the realisation of how many resources we lack compared with those in western countries. However, sometimes disadvantages can become advantages. For instance, not having intermediary structures such as group homes can be turned into an advantage by thinking about how to use existing services for 'normals' to create 'integrated' services. Lack of professionalism can be turned into more easily achieved equalitarian relationships with users, since Slovenia has a problem of imbalance between the well-developed profession of (hospital) psychiatry and under developed professions of social work and community psychiatric nursing.

Social work practitioners in Slovenia face a major challenge: how to gain influence as a profession and yet still remain close to the everyday life of the those we serve.

References

Basaglia, F. (1981) *Negacija institucije*, Beograd: Vidici br.5.

Basaglia, F. (1987) *Psychiatry Inside Out: Selected Works of Franco Basaglia, European Perspectives*, Columbia University Press.

Bion, W.R. (1963) *Experiences in Groups*, London: Tavistock.

Brandon D. (1991) *Innovation Without Change - Consumer involvement in psychiatric services*, London: Macmillan.

Brandon D. and Brandon A. (1991) *Staff Practice Handbook - a guide to practice in services for people with learning difficulties*, University College.

Salford; Slovene translation (1992) *Prakticni prirocnik za delo z ljudmi s posebnimi potrebami*, Ljubljana: VSSD & PEF.

Germain, Carol Bailey (1984) *Social Work Practice in Health Care*, London: Free Press.

Carlton, T.O. (1984) *Clinical Social Work in Health Care* Settings, New York: Springer.

Castel, R. (1976) *L'ordre psychiatrique*, Paris: Minuit.

Coulshed V. (1990) *Management in Social Work*, London: Macmillan.

de Board, R. (1978) *Psychoanalysis of Organisation*, London: Tavistock.

Freire, P. (1972) *Pedagogy of the Oppressed*, Penguin Books.

Goffman, E. (1961) *Asylums*, Doubleday & Co. (Pelican edition 1968).

Goffman E. (1963) *Stigma – Notes on the management of Spoiled Identity*, Engelwood Cliffs: Prentice-Hall (Penguin edition 1968).

Guattari, F. (1972) *Psychanalyse et transersalite*, Paris: Maspero.

Guattari, F. (1984) *Molecular Revolution*, Penguin Books.

Hughman, R. (1991) *Power in Caring Professions*, London: Macmillan.

Huxley, P. (1991) Social Work, in Bennet D.H. and Freeman H.L. *Community Psychiatry*, Edinburgh: Churchill Livingstone.

Jordan, B. (1984) *Invitation to Social Work*, Oxford, Basil Blackwell.

Jordan, B. (1987) Counselling, Advocacy and Negotiation *British Journal of Social Work* Vol. 17, N 2 (April 1987), pp. 135-146.

Øvretveit, J. (1993) *Coordinating Community Care - Multidisciplinary teams and care management*, Buckingam: Open University Press.

Payne, M. (1982) *Working in Teams*, London: Macmillan.

Ramon, S. and Giannichedda, M.G. (eds.) (1988) *Psychiatry in Transition*, London: Pluto Press.

Rose, S. and Black, B. (1985) *Advocacy and Empowerment: Mental Health Care in Community*, London: Routledge & Kegan Paul.

Scull, A. (ed.) (1981) *Madhouses Mad-Doctors and Madmen: The Social History of Psychiatry in Victorian Era*, London: The Athlone Press.

Southgate, J. and Randall, R. (1980) *Cooperative and Community Group Dynamics*, London: Barefoot Books.

Tilbury, D. (1993) Working with Mental Illness, London: Macmillan.

Chapter 9
Social Work Practice with Refugee Populations in Hungary: Process and Issues

Katalin Talyigas

Introduction

Dealing with refugees creates new professional and personal expectations and tasks for the social worker. The challenge is to help refugees move from problems of mere survival to the establishment of a brand-new life in a new and sometimes hostile environment.

Increasingly, those social workers involved in such activities are themselves part of a family history of flight and relocation. For example, the author's parents fled to Bolivia in 1938 because of the Nazis. After returning to Hungary following the Second World War, they were never able to forget their years in exile. I married a Bolivian citizen who himself had to run from his country in the 1960s because of political changes there. When the political winds changed again, he might have returned to his country, but he died in exile. This chapter is dedicated to all those who, having experienced it themselves, now try to ease the pain and suffering of those currently experiencing this process.

History of the Refugee Problem in Hungary

In spite of different situations in different countries, there are some common characteristics and challenges social workers face when serving refugee populations. Hungary's experience highlights some of them.

In eastern and central Europe there are some basic problems that have historical roots and affect contemporary life: (1) because the bourgeois of this region did not develop in the classical way, modernisation and economic development have been very slow; (2) the borders of the eastern and central European countries were formed according to political interests and ethnic background was not considered. There were waves of migration in this century: around 1900, between 1929 and 1933, after the Second World War, and especially in 1956. These migrations were for political, ethnic and economic reasons.

In 1989, the change of regimes in the east European Communist countries and the resulting economic crisis caused ethnic unrest. This changed Hungary from an emigratory country to an immigratory country. Refugees from Transylvania, from the former Yugoslavia and the former German Democratic Republic arrived in

Hungary. Some of them used Hungary as a temporary place on their way to western countries but a huge number of refugees have now lived in Hungary for years. The first refugees from Transylvania, 80-90 per cent of them minority Hungarians, came to Hungary in 1987. Political leaders responded to political pressure to officially support these refugees. Later an invasion by German Democratic Republic refugees trying to get to west Germany caused a problem. This was brilliantly resolved by the government; they removed the border fence separating the two political systems and permitted potential refugees to cross into west Germany.

A very dramatic change occured at the outbreak of the Yugoslav civil war when in a very short time Hungary faced the problem of servicing a great influx of refugees with different ethnic backgrounds. The refugees included Croatians, Serbs, Slovenians, Bosnians, Albanians and Russians. Most of them did not know Hungarian. They did not want to settle in Hungary but wished to return to their home or to emigrate to western countries.

Since 1989 two changes occurred. First, Hungary joined the Geneva Agreement on Refugee Affairs and began to establish the legal rules and institutions governing refugee affairs. Second, the economic conditions in Hungary changed and there was a substantial increase in unemployment. Hungarian people were threatened, afraid of losing their work and income. In the light of this threat, society's attitude toward the refugees changed. This caused ethnic conflicts even toward Hungarian minority refugees. Nationalism and the protection of Hungary's interest became one of the government's major political issues.

With the exception of a few charitable organisations Hungarian civil society's supportive interest in the refugee situation has ceased, even though by the end of 1991 Hungary had received more than 100,000 refugees who represented approximately one per cent of Hungary's inhabitants. The social welfare network operating in Hungary is not prepared to provide for the needs of these refugees. There is a lack of experts and financial resources. There are other deficiencies in the welfare system, such as lack of co-ordination between official government and civil or charitable organisations who deal with these issues. Also, the refugees' chance for employment and self-sufficiency has decreased.

Presently there are approximately 20,000 refugees living in Hungary. They have differing legal status. A few people have temporary permission to stay in Hungary, the first phase of immigration. Others are treated as 'conventional' refugees by the Geneva Convention, which gives them almost as many rights as Hungarian citizens.

However, most of the remaining 11,000 have only temporary 'fugitive' status. This means: (1) they get a 'fugitive identity card' that provides accommodation and food in a refugee camp or a 1,000 Ft/week (ten US dollars) contribution outside the camp, basic health care services and education; (2) they cannot work; (3) they cannot ask for social services from the municipalities or the National Welfare; (4) they cannot get a Hungarian or a 'conventional' passport; (5) they must return to the country they have escaped from to acquire official documents.

The reasons for these distinctions can be traced to the political will of a government whose policies are greatly constrained by a bad economic situation.

The problems of a refugee begin with authorities at the border. If the refugee enters the country at an official check-point, the refugee has to face the problem of being considered an 'economic immigrant'. Economic immigrants do not have normal passports and lack the amount of currency needed for entry as a tourist. Under these conditions the refugee is returned home.

However, there are situations where the refugee is successful in explaining the situation to the border guard. These refugees will be directed first to the special border surveillance officers and then to authorities of the Refugee Office of the Ministry of Interior. These officials decide the individual's status after completing an information form and conducting a short interview with the potential refugee.

Yugoslav refugees are usually classified as 'fugitives' and they are regulated only by one of the Ministry of Interior's Inner Directives, lacking even formal state administrative procedures. This puts these refugees in a defenceless position. They have to convince police officers that they are not 'economic immigrants' but are 'fugitives' escaping persecution. If approved as 'fugitives', they receive a short-term identity card allowing them to go to relatives, rent a flat if they have the resources to do so, or go to a refugee camp where they are submitted to a quarantine and an examination by the National Security Office.

The life experiences of refugees entering camps and of those able to survive dislocation by remaining outside the camps are very different and we shall examine those differences in detail.

Social Problems in the Nagyatad Refugee Camp[1]

This camp is located on the site of a former Soviet army base. The authority in charge of the camp is the Refugee Office of the Ministry of Interior, an arm of the military. Social workers are also responsible to this ministry. The primary role of the social worker in the camp is to pay personal attention to and meet individual needs of the refugees.

General Living Conditions. There are a lot of psychological and social problems among the refugees caused partly by the war which forced them to leave their friends, family members and their country, and partly by the conditions in the refugee camp.

Physical Conditions. First of all, refugees are surrounded by barbed wire and concrete walls, guarded by policemen and dogs, and have to beg permission to leave the facility even for a walk to the town. Many feel hopeless, like a long-term prisoner, because of their war experiences.

The physical space does not meet the needs of children, elderly people, or families. There is a *lack of privacy*. Children, and couples who have no opportunity for intimacy, and old people with sleep disturbances, all live together in a room with 20-30 other people. In the bathrooms, the shower stalls are not separated. This is especially disturbing to observant Muslims. Forty or more people share one bathroom. Most of the toilets do not function properly and though the refugees try to keep them clean, they are rarely provided with disinfectant to prevent sanitary problems. Everything is in need of repair and renovation. The stairs and floors are terribly dangerous when wet. Each room is heated with an enormous oil heater that has to be refilled daily during the winter. The oil exudes fumes, is a fire hazard and presents a danger to children.

Refugees have no control over the food served. It is high in fat content and low in nutritional value. There are Bosnian refugees employed in the kitchen but they are never consulted on issues of food selection, purchase or preparation. Food and other supplies for babies are sometimes in short supply. This gives parents a terrible feeling of not being able to provide for their children.

There is a hospital on the site as well as a home for the elderly, but there are sanitary problems and Hungarian health regulations do not deal with them.

All these aspects of the residents' lives affect how they feel about themselves and their surroundings. They do their best to make their living spaces as pleasant as possible, but living in conditions which they cannot control adds to their feeling of helplessness. Meanwhile, authorities in the camp and in Budapest openly admit that their policy is not to make the situation 'too good' for that might encourage the refugees to remain in Hungary.

Communication. The authorities and the residents themselves struggle with communication problems stemming from the fact that they speak different languages. Ethnic Hungarians are often employed as interpreters but are not trained to work with the refugees as social workers or interpreters. Though this employment of ethnic Hungarians is a practical use of resources, often there are miscommunications and arguments stemming from faulty translations. This provides another reason for the Bosnian refugees to feel a loss of control.

Almost all of the Hungarian residents of the camp are employed — either inside or outside the camp. It is clear that this is possible because of their language ability. This allows them privileges that the Bosnians do not have: more freedom, better living arrangements, respectful treatment from the staff, access to jobs and education, a chance for a future in Hungary. This often leads to conflict between Hungarian-speaking and non-Hungarian-speaking refugees that goes far beyond the problems that a *language barrier* would normally create.

Another communication problem in the camp stems from intolerance and impatience. The staff, including those providing social services, security guards, police and others in direct contact with the Bosnians are pervasively impatient, intolerant, and even rude to the refugees. The refugees feel this lack of common courtesy so strongly that they have lost all hope of their right to anything except a 'shelter' in Hungary. The situation is made worse by the consistent humiliating situations in which refugees are unnecessarily degraded. For example, staff members march into the rooms of the residents without knocking, uninvited and without formalities to demand some information or documentation, sometimes even without a translator.

The refugees are not correctly informed — or informed at the last-minute about something which will change their lives for ever. They do not have the opportunity to buy telephone cards necessary to make enquiries of the authorities or to phone their family in Bosnia. Although there is a committee of refugees which is consulted on certain issues, they actually have *very little influence to change things*. The refugees are afraid to speak up and many have lost hope of ever having any influence over their lives at Nagyatad.

Helplessness and Psychological Problems. The present situation in the camp is bounded by the *uncertainty* and *defencelessness* that people feel. They do not know if they will ever return home again; they do not have contacts with relatives and friends still in Bosnia; they do not have any hope, as far as they can see, for the future. Many men suffer guilt from not fighting for their country and sometimes there are physical confrontations. There are some refugees in the camp who were formerly imprisoned for illegal activities elsewhere in Europe, especially in Austria and Germany, and then deported. The refugees feel very insecure in the presence of these people. Also, people who 'misbehave' often get 'punishment' more severe than those who really do harm. Refugees then have the impression that camp authorities hold authority over issues of justice, and this makes them feel even more dependent.

The camp lacks trained psychologists and social workers. There is no one to simply sit and listen to the refugees or to advise and encourage them. For nine months there was a Bosnian refugee social worker brought to the camp by a German organisation. Her job was overwhelming. The residents came to her with all kinds of problems, from psychological distress to immigration issues. There are people called social workers who have never been trained as such in each of the refugees' residential buildings but they are too busy with administrative work to spend time with refugees or to give them personal attention, even should they wish to do so. These 'social workers' are not able to help with family reunification affairs or filling in foreign immigration forms, which could be a solution for many refugees, because they do not speak the necessary languages. Most of the staff involved with the higher levels of administration of the camp rarely enter the refugees' residential buildings. There is little chance for communication or developing understanding. Refugees in the camp are not permitted to call for a priest and as a result there have already been several suicide attempts.

Family structures are radically altered. Parents feel no longer truly responsible for taking care of their children and the children are involved in all aspects of life. This distorts parent:child communications. Many of the children amuse themselves violently, for example, playing 'war games'. A large number of children up to ten years of age wet their beds at night.

Elderly people in the camp suffer a different, unique kind of pain. Those who are relatively healthy live in the residential buildings with other refugees. Those who need constant medical care live in a separate home for the aged on the site. The elderly refugees feel that, unlike the younger refugees who sometimes feel a little hope, there will be no future for them. Many of them had never been outside their towns before the war and suddenly they find themselves in a refugee camp. The situation forces reconsideration of family ties and different ways of communicating within the family. Old people die at an unusually high rate not only because of the lack of adequate care and nutrition but because of trauma and anxiety related to changes in family structure and communication. It seems the greatest pain is due to their feeling that the younger members of their families may give up their own opportunities in order not to leave them behind. Many elderly people die earlier than they would if they were at home.

Existing Programmes. Children aged five to fourteen attend school in the camp. The large number of children attending makes it difficult for teachers to provide individual attention. During the summer months they are taken on rotation trips to Lake Balaton. Because they have these activities, they are perhaps relatively the least 'needy' group in the camp. One thing they do lack is personal attention. Their parents are often concerned with the family left in Bosnia or with issues of immigration. In many cases, children are left alone to play for long stretches of time.

For over a year, a group of Americans living and working in Budapest ('Friends of Nagyatad', started by Max Marcus) visited the children one week-end every six weeks. They carried out creative and sports programmes with the children. These trips were very successful, bonds of friendship were created and the children looked forward to the meetings with great excitement. Suddenly, for several months authorities denied the volunteers permission to enter the Nagyatad camp. The children felt yet again that they were forgotten.

Youngsters in the camp aged fourteen to twenty have absolutely no possibility of education. However, through the efforts of International Rescue Committee volunteers, teenagers have been involved in several programmes of theatre, basketball and weight-lifting, which helped release their accumulated physical and emotional energies. There were also language and music lessons, a Serb-Croatian library run by the refugees, excursions, handicraft projects, and summer trips to Lake Balaton. Those youngsters who learnt English have aided the volunteers and do interpreting and filling in immigration forms. However, only some of the young people participate in these programmes. Many others take a non-participatory attitude, often because they have not been able to deal with the trauma of their war experiences. They are the most 'needy' group and the least likely to ask for help.

Women in the camp are in need of support. The uncertain situation causes personal and family problems which impinge on them constantly. The Handicrafts Project and sewing projects run by the International Rescue Committee activists have provided over 300 women an occupational activity and a considerable amount of income but the camp authorities do nothing to aid the project.

Men suffer from unemployment although there are skilled workers whom the Hungarian authorities could use instead of Hungarian workers. The unemployment causes nervousness, restlessness and arguments.

There are a few positive changes. For example, observant Muslims now have access to menus which respect their cultural diet. Some refugees have been able to move to another country or find a job in Hungary with the help of the American volunteers. Still, the needs of the refugees by far exceed these opportunities.

The Situation of Refugees Outside the Camps

Refugees outside camps are in a much better position than those inside. Many had friends or relatives in Hungary who helped them find free boarding during the first wave of refugees, when villages near the border accepted them. Although the attitude of civil society has become less receptive, refugee families in this situation can still live a better life and have more freedom.

However, this 'free' life means that refugees have to provide themselves with everything they need and cover all living costs. Their only help is a 1,000 FT/week/person (equal to ten US dollars) contribution from the authorities until they get a regular job, and sometimes a food or clothes pack from a charitable organisation.

Most of these refugee people have 'fugitive' status and cannot apply for a 'regular' job. They have to take on 'black' work, work that they would not be willing to do in normal circumstances. They receive the same free medical care as local residents although the refugee population often suffers from the results of under-feeding and under-heating due to the costs; and, like village residents, may not get special health services for some chronic illnesses. They have schools in their own language and learn Hungarian as a second language. These refugees can therefore integrate somewhat into local society.

Harkany is an example of this. It is a village of 4,000 inhabitants which took on 8,000 worn out refugees during the first wave. It has two district physicians and two nurses that serve the entire village. The municipality, the Red Cross and other sponsors contributed to the residents who lodged and fed the refugees for many months. These refugees assumed they would return to their homes soon. At the end of six months, however, they realised they had to create a more stable position in Hungary as it was evident the war would not soon end. By this time, the reserves of both the boarding families and the refugees had decreased. Still, there were no serious problems and with the help of village residents refugees found places to stay, sometimes at their own expense. When they realised the need, the refugees somehow acquired the necessary resources. For example, through personal acquaintances they found more or less stable jobs, mobilised their reserves in Bosnia, or asked for money from relatives in Germany. These families have now been able to sustain themselves for as long as three years. They have natural helpers whom they trust, for example neighbours, relatives, priest and doctor.

B.D. serves as an example. She is a Hungarian woman who escaped from Serbia with her son three years ago. A teacher by profession and able to speak both Hungarian and Serbian, she quickly found a job in the school for the refugees.

This entitles her to all welfare services. She found a flat in the home of a friend where she pays only the running costs so she is in a favourable situation. Her husband refuses to join her and she faces the dilemma of what to say and how to behave so that her son, who still loves his father, does not get psychologically hurt because his father has found another woman. Women usually do not discuss these situations but many of them have given up being a 'woman' in order to remain 'a good mother'. Such problems affected B.D. so much that she contacted a social worker via whom her health problems were diagnosed. Placement of a pacemaker was necessary to stabilise her heart.

It is useful to draw this rough comparison between 'camp' life and 'free' life because both refugees and social workers face somewhat different tasks and have different experiences.

Implications for Social Work: Basic Principles

To effectively serve these refugees, social workers must know specifically the legal environment, the social context and the experience of day-to-day living for all segments of this population. They must also know the psychological and cognitive aspects of refugee life. Of special importance is how refugees have dealt with the crisis of relocation, the circumstances they suffered before leaving their home of origin, the 'unfinished business' left behind (such as relatives, property, business interests, and friends).

There are economic, social and cultural factors which strongly influence refugees' behaviour, their decision making and the way they wish to be treated. First, they suffer deeply from feelings of being victims of 'power games'. They came from a country where they could have been sacked from their jobs simply because of their nationality, put out of their houses by local authorities or soldiers, or even had a knife put to their throats. Until the war, people in Yugoslavia did not pay much attention to their nationality. Now they have learnt what political and military powers, any kind of authority, can do to their families. They never talk about their fear and anger and they trust only themselves and their family.

There are also examples of 'mishelp' in regard to the expatriates, which leave more impressions of the misuse of power. This leads to a maximum avoidance of asking for help. For example, Bosnian mothers lost interest in feeding their own babies when they were told that they neglected the children and were instructed on how they should care for them. The women then simply left this task of caring for the children to the surprised social worker! Also, pregnant women were often told to have an abortion.

Another example of 'mishelp' is the present policy of Hungarian authorities and charitable organisations to establish an 'old age' home for elderly refugees, even though not a single Bosnian family agreed with this solution. Despite all their burdens, the Bosnians would rather see contributions of medicines or help from a nurse instead of what they perceive as 'throwing out' the elderly.

Refugees also have an impression that they are 'second rate people' in the host country and have to be 'quiet' during their stay there. Therefore a social worker needs to do everything possible to help the refugee gain positive impressions about the host country.

Another influence on the refugees' psychology is economic dependence. Most of these people previously had a middle class existence and had no need to rely on the help of the state, family or friends. Suddenly they had to leave all their belongings, start a new, poor life in a foreign country, often only with the 'possibilities' a camp can offer. They say: 'We don't need state support, give us an opportunity to work!'

These people feel they are deprived of the right to decide upon their privacy by the authorities and the 'social workers'. These factors often lead to apathy, depression, the disorganisation of social ties generally, and the total separation of emotional ties between members of families and other individuals. This begins a process which is very hard to stop.

Considering these factors in each case, a social worker must be very patient and understanding and take effective measures in the interests of the refugees in order to gain their trust. This is the first, absolutely essential phase if a social worker is to gradually be able to help refugees.

It begins with the initiation of a contact. Refugees turn to the social worker very rarely, only in an extremely bad situation, so there is usually a major crisis by the time the refugee initiates contact. In this phase a social worker must consider the feelings of a refugee who must now receive help from a total stranger while existing in a poor living environment.

In usual practice, a good social worker does not go to the house of the client without an invitation, but the opposite recurrently happens in the camp. The best place to meet a refugee for the first time is in a neutral place such as one of the camp's community areas. It is also good to bring along, not only a person who speaks the language, but also a member of the refugee group or other reference person whom they trust. A female social worker must be very aware of how she dresses and behaves when she visits a Muslim family and be sure to observe customs such as taking off shoes, not drinking coffee, and not to look in a man's eye.

Social Work Practice with Refugee Populations in Hungary: Process and Issues

The next step is the engagement phase. At first, refugees do not see their situation clearly. They are not able to suggest realistic, long-term objectives. Usually they identify the most urgent and basic problems. This problem definition must be accepted by the social worker without reservations. The social worker cannot expect any help from the client, even if the client promises it, as the social worker has to 'prove' that things will change and achieve a tangible success in order to earn the trust of the client. This happens by small steps and the social worker must be very careful not to create false expectations or spoil the contact with confrontations. The social worker must respect confidentiality and seek agreement of the client to talk with relatives or neighbours as there may be disagreements on some issues. A social worker may practically deal with only four to five families during initial stages, but could work with fifteen to twenty families if there are no crisis situations.

The social worker also has to try to provide positive impressions about the host country during this phase. Examples would be to find some job where the refugee can meet Hungarian people in a good work-place atmosphere, or 'neighbours' who help him, or a school where his child can be with Hungarian children. This eases the feelings of defencelessness, of being the victims of power games, and improves the general feelings of comfort which can affect all aspects of everyday life.

After the development of trust, a real problem-solving process can start. It must be based on a chain of agreements between refugee and social worker and the proper exploration of the problems and hopes of the client. During initial contacts, there are such statements as: 'I would like to return home' and 'I wish this war never happened!' In fact, there is a process of re-experiencing the traumas of war. The social worker must give serious attention to this because the client usually cannot concentrate on practical issues until these events have been dealt with in some way. The client needs to talk about the trauma, to release part of the pressure, to share the meaning of the experience and to integrate the experience with his or her own life-course. The social worker must reflect these feelings with empathy and ascertain what kind of help the client will accept at this stage. The social worker who does not realise the importance of these steps is often not aware of the traumas that affect the thoughts and the dreams of the client. Until these steps are taken, work toward practical objectives, such as finding a job or locating a flat, will fail.

The social worker must be able to handle the outbreak of emotions such as crying, desperation and aggression at these vulnerable points and show real compassion, turning this drama into a relieving catharsis. During this time, the social worker has to possess empathy towards the client and try to be able to see the experience through the client's eyes. Both verbal and non-verbal communication are important components of the communication process at this stage.

Only after some of this work has been done can the social worker and client agree on the action plan for the solution of a problem and begin its implementation. A main principle is that the social worker should believe in the client and the individual's problem-solving abilities. Worker and client should jointly acknowledge the points where decisions must be made that will help manage changes in the 'outside world' and effect some solution to the problem identified.

The social worker has to be able to provide correct information about the possibilities in the host country and draw a realistic picture of the refugee's new environment. In this planning process, the social worker can share professional experience and knowledge and point out the potential impact of available options on the client and on others. But mostly the social worker looks to the will of the client. The social worker becomes a 'tool' to help the client reach his goals.

In implementation of the plan, accomplishment of small steps helps refugees feel that individually (or together with the family) there has been success in something. They will then agree to do things they would prefer not to do, but which are necessary, to reach their goal or solve their problem. For example, refugees will start to attend a language course if they feel that this is what they need to do to find a job. Often tasks can be divided. For example, the social worker can say what documents are needed for a work permit and the client can bring them so that work can proceed. They will then work together to find an employer. The social worker must know current local circumstances, have a network of local sources of information, and know the legal 'tricks' that help find jobs for refugees.

The parting or terminating phase of the process is often not handled well. Usually by the end of their work together, having reached a goal or solved a problem, something like a 'good acquaintanceship' develops and the social worker is seen as a person who can be trusted and one who understands. The social worker must realise that a social worker functions as an 'artificial helper' who has done a good job if the client manages to change the situation and, as a result of the experience, is better equipped to solve future problems without professional intervention or dependency. The social worker should gradually prepare the client for this emotional parting although leaving the door open for occasional meetings should future problems arise.

Implications for Professional Social Work
There are essential qualities needed when dealing directly with refugees:
- respect for the personality and privacy of the client;
- empathy and patience;

- thorough knowledge of customs and norms of the past and present community of the client;
- lack of prejudices of any kind, no distinctions between those who 'deserve' help and those who don't;
- ability to gradually enable clients to solve problems themselves;
- ability to help integration into the local society.

In Hungary, the role of the social worker with regard to refugee populations is currently limited to work with individual refugees, provided mainly by volunteers. If a systems approach were employed to analyse refugee problems and the contributions social work could make to solving them, other professional contributions would be highlighted. Provisions could be made in the camps for in-service training which would heighten sensitivities of staff; group work could help severely depressed parents and children with behavioural problems. Advocacy and small group work activities could strengthen the role of the resident councils in creating more freedom and better living conditions in the camp, and help refugees establish some feeling of control over their lives. The refugees' motivation could then be directed to making a life-plan for leaving.

In communities, social workers could foster development strategies which address the needs of refugees as a special population rather than as individuals.

Currently, even work with individual refugees is episodic. There is no plan to deal with continuing problems of loss and grief, anger and hostility, the continuing need for social support and the long-range effects of trauma and displacement.

Development of a system which meets these needs will require dedicated attention and sanction from authorities and the advocacy and planning skills of social workers and others. One or two professionally trained social workers, used at the policy level of government, or even at the level of the camp, might be hired to examine the impact of existing policies and to recommend changes; goals would be to reduce long-time dependency and despondency which would create problems and costs in the future.

In terms of families, social work intervention could help stabilise family structure and communication and decision making, helping maintain the cohesion necessary to keep families intact and the family support system as a facilitative structure which promotes growth and integration into society.

Social work interventions, such as group work, can help families cope with their children's anger and anxiety in a way which fosters normal development in children and may also prevent child abuse.

Refugees may be able to learn to use the camp environment as one for learning group decision making, leadership and advocacy skills with the help of professionally trained social workers.

The humanistic value base of the profession would dictate that social work services be directed to development of a humane living environment and relieving the existential pain, as well as the physical hardship, endured by these hapless victims. The necessity for understanding, acknowledging and respecting the historical and cultural backgrounds from which refugees originate and to which they flee cannot be overestimated.

Even if professional social work services are made available to the expatriates, they will seek access to them and utilise them only if the services are perceived to be viable within their ethnic/cultural context and if they are provided by social workers sensitive to ethnic/cultural concerns. This demands that social workers put aside personal prejudices and perhaps overlook negative historical or cultural experiences in their own personal lives in order to serve this population in a professional manner. That is the challenge to the profession, individually and collectively.

The Social Work School of Szeged Medical University has started a course on social work with refugees. The Hungarian Red Cross and the Geneva Agency currently hold extensive seminars especially for those who work in refugee affairs. This improved training should lead to better conditions and services that will contribute to a more humane existence for these traumatised and displaced populations.

Notes
1   Based on material from Max Marcus, American RCI Volunteer, Nagyatad.

References
Based on material from Max Marcus, American volunteer with the International Rescue Committee (RCI) and material from Kovacs V. Ilona, social worker dealing with refugees, and from Forral Sando, volunteer.

Toth, Judity: *Refugees in Hungary*; pub. Akademia (in Hungarian).

Sik, Endre; *Statistics on Refugees: Studies of Nagy Boldizsar and Kovacs* Vl. Ilona.

Introduction to the Empowerment Framework Exemplars

A humane society emphasises opportunities for its members to fully participate in the civil and social life of the community. A humane health care system emphasises and facilitates people's adoption of community social roles rather than sick roles which foster dependence and isolation.

It is in performance of their social roles in the ordinary life of the community that people have opportunities for social relationships which are the essence of being fully human. They have the opportunity to express feelings, enjoy sources of emotional support, and gain satisfaction by meeting the expectations of others and of themselves. Performance of social roles helps people gain information on which to base their sense of reality, make some assessment about their future, and learn about the resources offered by their community.

Those who are chronically ill or disabled have historically been deprived of the opportunity to fully participate in the life of the community. This deprivation has occurred because they were isolated in large hospitals and institutions, denied access to environments by physical barriers (such as stairs) or forced by the public's attitudes to abandon participation in the life of the community.

A government's role in providing this type of humane environment and humane health care for the people it governs varies in countries throughout the world and at different times within the same country. Governments in Britain and the United States have assumed some responsibility for health care over the last 100 years. In east European and former Communist countries government dictated design of a centralised, heavily bureaucratised medical system. Progressive socialist countries such as Norway and Sweden pioneered in deinstitutionalisation and providing community care and integration.

The following two chapters present insights into changing patterns of care in the United States and the United Kingdom and examine how social work practitioners are facilitating these changes. Chapter 10 provides an evolutionary perspective on the move toward community living and away from institutionalisation in the United States since the 1940s. These changes have been encouraged by larger changes in society, such as the civil rights movement, which brought about significant policy changes at the national level that impact on the quality of life of those with disabilities. In this sense, the chapter presents somewhat of a 'top down' perspective.

Chapter 11 provides an insight into changes in the self-definition and stance of many of those in the United Kingdom who have chronic illnesses and/or disabling conditions. They refuse to be set aside, refuse to be isolated from the community and they actively advocate for the resources they need to fully participate in an ordinary way of life. By working individually and with groups, and by designing and facilitating interventions at various levels, social workers can behave in ways that facilitate integration and participation in community life by those who might otherwise be excluded. Chapter 11 presents a 'bottom to top' approach to social work practice that is committed to people empowerment, helping people realise their own power, solve their own problems and take control of their own lives.

Both chapters indicate that social workers must focus on strengths, not deficiencies, of the people they serve. Both chapters subscribe to the thesis that the goal of social work is to help clients exert power in a way that enables them to obtain the resources necessary to meet their needs, both individually and collectively. Both focus their practice interventions on the person:environment interface.

Power is a central component in both these chapters. Power is a necessary commodity for people who desire to achieve some control over their destiny. Social workers can practise in a way that fosters this development of power and removes barriers that diminish opportunities to achieve power. Both chapters focus on a model of social work practice which (1) helps people gain the capacity to counteract the negative forces which affect their lives, (2) helps them confront social situations which are oppressive and distort their psychological well-being, and (3) helps people gain control over these situations (Pinderhughes, 1983).

Both policy-makers and clinicians recognise that 'to focus on client strengths and to practise with the intent of client empowerment is to practise with an explicit power consciousness ... Assessing specific obstacles to empowerment, assessing power relationships, and assessing the relationship between personal empowerment and social empowerment of the individual' are identified as assessment issues for those working within an empowerment framework (Cowger, 1994). Because its focus is power, those practising most intensely within this framework are working in a politically charged arena which sometimes requires faith and sacrifice on the part of both workers and clients. Changing the balance of power in relationships — individually, collectively and internationally — is fraught with conflict even though it results in constructive change.

Introduction to the Empowerment Framework Exemplar

The experiences of everyday life, and of everyday social work practice, should inform social policies which affect the social fabric of daily life. As such, public policy reflects an evolutionary process that at any given moment is the result of a given society's reflections on its past and a projection of its future.

The future consists in learning from the past as well as from the utilisation of emerging technologies and predictions about the future. These two chapters focus on past, present and future. To learn from the past, engage in the present and help form the future, social workers need to be effective communicators as individual practitioners. They must also be visible and influential through their professional organisations if they are to contribute to the social policies that will govern the future.

They need to be part of the voice that is heard by those formulating public policies that could either diminish or empower those who risk being kept at the margins of society.

References

Cowger, C.D.; Assessing Client Strengths: Clinical Assessment for Client Empowerment; Social Work; *Journal National Association of Social Workers*, Vol 39 issue 3; May, 1994 Wash. D.C.

Pinderhughes, Elaine B.; Empowerment for Our Clients and Ourselves; *Social Casework*, Vol. 64; June 1983.

Chapter 10
Social Work Practice Among Individuals with Disabling Conditions: An Evolutionary Perspective

Mariellen Laucht Kuehn and John W. McClain

Introduction

Over the past sixty years, the service and support systems for individuals with disabling conditions in the United States have evolved from institutional living to community integration. The move to community integration for individuals with disabilities has been relatively fast and relates directly to shifts in social values and technological advances that have occurred during the twentieth century. Today individuals with disabilities are viewed as full citizens participating in a democratic society who are capable of living productive, independent lives within their own culture and the community of their choice. The intent of this chapter is to provide an historical and evolutionary perspective on the issues and concerns of individuals with disabling conditions and their families and the role of social workers who serve and support them.

Definitions

For decades, efforts have been made to construct diagnostic classification systems for diseases and mental health conditions which are often noted as biologically based disease entities. The purpose of medical classifications has been to systematically study the aetiology, prevention and treatment of disease in order to establish standardised plans for diagnosis and treatment.

Definitions and Disabling Conditions. Classifications are considered helpful for professionals working with individuals with disabilities as they can be used to determine the most valid procedures for assessment, intervention and case management. The primary disadvantage of these classification systems is that individuals are often labelled and negatively valued by society on the basis of a classification. As a result of such labelling, individuals often are stereotyped, discriminated against, and restricted by social attitudes or policies. Although classification systems do not account for individual variations in culture or biology, they are used extensively by social workers and other service professionals to determine appropriate standardised assessment and intervention plans. They also may be used by policymakers to determine a person's eligibility for public financial assistance and services.

Within the United States today, children and young adults (individuals under age 22) with disabilities are generally classified as having a *chronic handicapping condition or a developmental disability*. Chronic handicapping conditions are primarily medical disabilities, such as juvenile diabetes, cancer, AIDS, haemophilia, pulmonary or respiratory disease (such as cystic fibrosis), heart conditions and arthritis. Children with emotional disorders, such as depression or schizophrenia, also are categorised as having a chronic handicapping condition. Children with chronic handicapping conditions usually need ongoing and continuous medical care and treatment, including regular hospital visits, to support and maintain their lives. Since for these children survival is frequently a primary concern, medical care often takes precedence over a child's social, economic and/or cultural needs.

Children with *developmental disabilities* have conditions which affect their cognitive and/or physical (motor, hearing, visual, speech and/or language) development and limit their functional capabilities. Examples of developmental disabilities include: cognitive disorders such as Down syndrome, mental retardation and autism; neurological disorders such as cerebral palsy; genetic disorders such as dwarfism; metabolic disorders such as phenylketonuria (PKU) and galactosemia; and accidental injury that has caused brain trauma or physical disabilities such as spinal cord injury. Children with developmental disabilities may or may not experience emotional difficulties. Those with developmental disabilities usually are dependent upon the knowledge and skills of an interdisciplinary team of professionals that includes social workers. These interdisciplinary teams work together with family members to maintain and/or improve the functional capabilities of children and to support their integration within their home, school and community.

Adults with disabilities include individuals who have aged chronologically and were born with a chronic handicapping condition or a developmental disability. Adults with disabilities also include individuals who have a chronic medical (physical or mental) condition that began later in life and is most likely to continue throughout the lifespan, such as adult on-set diabetes, multiple sclerosis, Parkinson's disease, arthritis, schizophrenia or Alzheimer's. Other adults with disabilities have become disabled as the result of an accidental injury or trauma due to such events as an automobile accident or a heart attack.

Most individuals with disabling conditions are classified by one or more medical or psychological diagnoses based upon the International Classification of Diseases Tenth Revision Clinical Modification (ICD-10-CM) or the Diagnostic and Statistical Manual of Mental Disorders, Fourth Edition (DSM-IV).

Social Work Practice Among Individuals with Disabling Conditions: An Evolutionary Perspective

Individuals with disabling conditions, particularly developmental disabilities, often are classified by categorical diagnoses as well as on the basis of specific physical, mental and/or functional characteristics. Hence, a person may be diagnosed as having a mental disorder (ICD9-CM 317-318) and/or categorically as having Down syndrome. Social workers who provide services to individuals with disabling conditions need to be conversant with these classification systems in order to work effectively in multidisciplinary settings such as hospitals, clinics and institutions.

Implications for Social Work Practice. The view of disabling conditions and individuals with disabilities has radically evolved over the past 30 years from one primarily grounded in the medical aetiology of a particular disease to a view which focuses upon the unique social and psychological impact of disability on the life of an individual. This broader view integrates medical classifications and medical/health concerns. It also examines an individual's capacity to function (provide self-care and interact in a community environment) within a holistic framework that integrates the biological, psychological and social aspects of the human experience. This approach permits social workers to focus on the uniqueness of a particular client and to facilitate a comprehensive habilitation or rehabilitation plan for providing the supports and services needed by an individual with a disability and their family.

Because of the complexity of the problems facing most individuals with disabilities, there has been a movement away from an exclusive reliance on clinical diagnoses based upon medical aetiology to an approach based on comprehensive functional assessments conducted by social workers as part of an interdisciplinary team. Functional assessments permit the social worker to focus on the individual as a social creature, performing tasks which define that person as a member of a family and as a member of a broader community. Social workers, through the utilisation of functional assessments, must continually ask themselves what unique impact the physical and/or mental disabling condition has on an individual's ability to establish a meaningful role that is in harmony with the culture in which the individual is immersed. Functional assessments are at once liberating and humbling. They are liberating because of their ability to provide valuable guides for appropriate interventions. They are humbling because they force recognition of the multiple, complex and interwoven social, cultural and economic problems a person and his or her family must address.

A functional assessment is a comprehensive one of an individual and his or her levels of functioning. This allows a professional to identify the support and service needs of a person in major functional areas. The most common components of functional assessment are:

- physical health status including all diagnoses, medications, number of visits to a hospital or physician in the recent past and the reason for those visits, alcohol usage and smoking habits;
- impact of physical condition on motor and communication (hearing, visual, speech and language) abilities;
- mental health status including cognitive problem-solving capabilities and affective aspects such as worry and life satisfaction;
- activities of daily living including ability to care for his or her body functions (bathing, teeth brushing, hair combing and so forth) and ability to participate in societal (employment, leisure and community) activities;
- personal goals (educational, vocational, social and recreational) and lifestyle preferences (culture, community, style of dress, food preferences and so forth);
- capabilities and strengths of the individual which can be used for activities of daily living and for achieving his or her life goals and lifestyle preferences; and
- environmental barriers (physical and social) in the school, home and community to achieving his or her personal goals and lifestyle preferences;
- economic status and access to financial means of support;
- social support systems which provide both social and emotional supports and physical supports to assist with the daily living activities and to facilitate the accomplishment of the individual's personal goals and lifestyle preferences.

This shift in emphasis from a solely medical diagnosis to one involving functional assessment has established a route to professional equality for social workers who, for a long time, have been subordinated by the medical approach to problem solving and treatment regimens for individuals with disabilities. As a result of this shift, the social worker's traditional focus on psychosocial functioning, social supports and finding resources to meet individual and family needs has become more valued.

Social Work Practice Among Individuals with Disabling Conditions:
An Evolutionary Perspective

The following sections of this chapter provide a brief overview of the role of social workers serving people with disabilities in the context of changing social conditions throughout this century and the implications for social work practice in the future.

Social Work and Disabling Conditions — 1900 to 1940

This chapter's major focus is on the social context and the social work role after 1940, when care of those with disabling conditions shifted from institutions to the community. Between 1900 and 1940, however, there were developments which significantly influenced that shift:

- a transition from an agricultural to an industrial society;
- severe economic depression which forced re-examination of the belief that unemployment was the consequence of individual moral decay;
- emergence of a social philosophy that provided for government intervention when natural market forces generated economic chaos;
- economic relief, provided by the government, when an individual could document that their economic misfortune was generated by factors beyond their control.

In regard to the care of those with disabling conditions, this period saw the following developments:

- scientific advancements in the study of immunology and serology;
- the founding of public hospitals for children;
- establishment of the first hospital social work department, whose social workers were required to (a) report home and social conditions of the patient's life and (b) provide a linkage between the hospital and community agencies (Nacman, 1977);
- federally funded crippled children's services (including physician, dentistry, public health nursing, medical social work and nutrition services) and development of a nationwide network of clinics and programmes;
- federal funding for the training of professional social workers and medical personnel who would serve children with many types of disabling conditions.

Although children with chronic handicapping conditions were often born in children's hospitals, many died shortly after birth or during early childhood.

Those who survived received minimal medical care. Many were often viewed by families and communities as a sign of moral and physical decay — Divine retribution for some past transgression of family members.

Institutionalisation was viewed as the most humane approach to the care of such children since it protected families from harsh social scrutiny and from the physical and emotional burdens engendered by the care of such children. Thus families already burdened by profound grief, anger and anxiety frequently also faced a moral dilemma — to follow their own desires to preserve familial bonds, or to follow society's conventional wisdom and institutionalise their child. Many families chose to provide for their offspring within the family home. However, this provided both the child and the family with a circumscribed, isolated, and often stigmatised way of life. Social workers provided limited professional support for such families.

Social workers began incorporating psychoanalytic and behavioural theories into casework practice during this period, but individuals with developmental disabilities, such as mental retardation, were not served. Frequently families struggling with management and emotional issues regarding such family members were also not served.

A primary role for professional social workers during this time was the role of social activist/social change agent. Social workers were involved in political campaigns and efforts to improve milk supplies, housing, sanitation, child labour conditions, social health programmes, pure food and drug laws and social reform legislation that provided a 'safety net' to protect Americans from market forces outside their control.

As a result of other legislation, social workers also: (1) evolved into 'gatekeepers' for society; (2) provided welfare services for the poor and disabled; (3) conducted eligibility tests which determined whether a person would receive publicly funded financial assistance. Participation in such work often put social workers in a strategic position to identify structural problems within society and to promote additional social change.

All these social work activities from 1900 to 1940 exerted a positive influence on the general health and well-being of mothers and their children, but families of individuals with developmental disabilities and other disabling conditions continued to receive, at best, peripheral attention.

*Social Work Practice Among Individuals with Disabling Conditions:
An Evolutionary Perspective*

Social Work and Disabling Conditions — 1940 to 1970

In the years during and following the Second World War, there was a significant population explosion in the United States. There also was an increasing migration from the small rural communities in the country to the larger, developing urban centres. These changes resulted in a shortage of physicians, social workers, and other health care professionals to provide primary health care services and there was an increased demand for social welfare services and supports.

The Social Context from 1940 to 1970. During this period, there were many social and economic changes in the United States. The discovery of antibiotics and psychotropic drugs reduced childhood diseases and permitted the care of individuals with mental disabilities in the community as opposed to the institution. It was also a time of raised expectations for a secure future and a good life for everyone. Servicemen returning from the Second World War found themselves eligible for an array of rehabilitative services which addressed their war-generated physical and mental disabilities. They also were offered economic support to facilitate their integration into the new prosperity associated with the emergence of the United States as an economic leader in the world. As Americans looked forward to a boundless future, concerns for the inheritors of that future — the American children — were raised.

Optimism and faith in the future and the concerns for children were highlighted by a 1950 White House Conference which focused on the mental and emotional development of all children and included a highlighting of children with chronic handicapping conditions and developmental disabilities. As an outcome of this conference and other federal initiatives, the federal Maternal and Child Health Agency received additional funds to establish clinical demonstration programmes for children with mental retardation. As a result of this funding, first allocated in 1957, new diagnostic, consultative, and educational clinics were established nationwide. The goal of this legislation was to offer health and education services within the community for children with mental retardation and other cognitive disabilities. However, the majority of children with developmental disabilities continued to live in private, charitable or government-sponsored institutions.

Historically, institutions had been seen as temporary havens for individuals with developmental disabilities. Originally, the institutions were established to provide education and training before eventual release into the community. Institutions were hailed as therapeutic innovations. Unfortunately, the prejudices of society and the social problems associated with the frequent abandonment of individuals with disabilities by their families once they returned to the community altered the original intent of using institutions as temporary training centres. Instead, institutions became permanent residences for individuals with disabilities, particularly those with developmental disabilities.

Economic considerations had transformed relatively small institutions into large complexes that housed hundreds of individuals of all ages with all types of disabling conditions. These massive complexes were rigidly controlled, provided few services beyond minimal daily maintenance, and encouraged the abuses associated with institutions of this kind. The social philosophy of the period viewed individuals with disabilities as incapable of leading productive lives in the community and needing constant supervision to prevent their involvement in criminal activity and other immoral behaviour. Theoretically, institutions protected individuals with disabilities from the pitfalls and negative temptations of community life and, in turn, they protected society from the illicit behaviour associated with individuals with disabling conditions, particularly those individuals with mental retardation.

The decade of the 1960s saw a great deal of civil unrest in the United States and the civil rights movement was started. The seeds for this civil rights movement were, in part, sown during the Great Depression and the Second World War. The social philosophy which held that economic forces and social structures, rather than a person's immoral behaviour, contributed to the poverty of an individual remained intact. However, the rising expectations for a new world generated by African-American soldiers, who were exposed to a less-overtly-racist environment in Europe, generated a commitment to securing equal rights for all American citizens. This civil rights movement focused primarily on the concerns of African-Americans, but the movement later gave rise to a multiplicity of civil rights movements among such disenfranchised groups as women and adults who had a disabling condition. These demands for civil rights placed the emphasis on changing the social and economic structure and not upon the moral or other perceived defects of the individual.

It was within this social context that parents and other family members became increasingly concerned for the quality of life that their children in the institutions were experiencing. Initially, social reform efforts were aimed at normalising the environment within the institution (Wolfensberger, 1972). The idea was to replicate a normalising routine of life and a quality community life within the confines of the institution. It wasn't until later in the 1970s and early 1980s that social reform efforts shifted from normalisation of the institutional life to deinstitutionalisation and the return of individuals with developmental disabilities to society.

Social Work Practice Among Individuals with Disabling Conditions: An Evolutionary Perspective

The Role of Social Work from 1940 to 1970. During this time period, social workers continued to work in hospitals and in institutions, providing services to individuals with disabilities and their families. Within the hospital setting, the role of social worker included: the identification of patients and families requiring social work services, assessment of home environment factors which would influence the care and treatment of patients, evaluation and treatment of crisis situations, and discharge planning. Often, social workers, as part of their jobs, were required to assist families with locating and arranging for institutional care for their child who had a developmental disability.

The majority of social workers were slow to accept the rising concern for individuals with mental retardation and other developmental disabilities (Adams, 1971). There were a small number of social workers who, with support from their professional organisation and/or the institutions of higher education who were training professional social workers, did make significant contributions which have been summarised by Horejsi (1983). These included:

- individual and group counselling for those with mental retardation and their family members;
- social evaluations, as part of an interdisciplinary team;
- the development of alternative living arrangements, such as foster homes;
- the evolution of protective services;
- the provision of advocacy services to assist individuals with mental retardation and/or their families to obtain the services they need;
- availability of intake and discharge planning; and
- community organisation, social planning, and administrative activities.

Regardless of whether social workers were employed by hospitals, health care clinics, institutions or community service agencies, some social workers also began to experiment with modifying established psychotherapeutic and behavioural approaches to improve social work services for individuals with disabilities and their families. Other social workers were involved in political endeavours to increase the provision of services for with disabilities.

In 1961 President John F. Kennedy appointed a Panel on Mental Retardation that was attended by scientists, educators, social workers, and other individuals concerned with mental retardation. As a result of a conference, President Kennedy created the National Institute of Child Health and Human Development and the President's Committee on Mental Retardation. Some of the critical pieces of legislation which were passed as a result of these endeavours included legislation which:

- supported the expansion and improvement of the federal Crippled Children's Programmes to prevent and combat mental retardation (1963);
- provided grants to support the construction of research centres and for University Affiliated Facilities to serve individuals with mental retardation (1963); and
- provided funding for University Affiliated Facilities to train social workers and other health professionals to serve children with chronic handicapping conditions and their families (1965).

Social Work and Disabling Conditions — 1970 to the Present

During the period from 1970 to the present, there has been a continuing emphasis upon civil rights and social justice for all people regardless of race or ethnicity and for individuals with disabilities.

The Social Context from 1970 to the Present. It was in the context of the civil rights movements of the 1960s that the social conscience of the general public in the United States was aroused with regard to the needs of all individuals with disabling conditions. Within the social work profession, there was increased recognition that mental retardation (and other disabilities) was not a private tragedy but, rather, a social problem correlated with poverty and the lack of social policies to ensure safe environments for mothers and their children (Wikler & Berkowitz, 1983).

There was particular concern about those individuals with developmental disabilities who were placed in institutions. Placement in institutions was seen as depriving them of their right to the freedoms that all members of a democratic society have a right to expect. It was at this time that the movement toward deinstitutionalisation was born.

The deinstitutionalisation movement focused on the prevention of new admissions to institutions, the transfer of individuals with developmental disabilities to their home community, the establishment of service and support systems at the community level, and planning for the eventual closure of government-sponsored institutions.

Social Work Practice Among Individuals with Disabling Conditions: An Evolutionary Perspective

Advocacy efforts shifted from improving the quality of life in institutions toward the integration of individuals with developmental disabilities into the community at large. The families of individuals with developmental disabilities, social workers, and other health professionals expanded their recognition of the social environment as a critical component in the growth and development of children as efforts were initiated to transfer individuals from institutions to the community. Strategies were initiated to give recognition to the capabilities and capacity of individuals with developmental disabilities and others with serious disabling conditions to contribute to community life.

As a result of the advocacy efforts of the families of individuals with disabilities, social workers, lawyers and other professionals working on behalf of those individuals with disabling conditions, several pieces of critical legislation were passed to facilitate the deinstitutionalisation process. For example, legislation was passed in 1973 which prohibits discrimination on the basis of disability in any federal programme, and in 1975 an amendment to the Social Security Act was passed that provided an array of social services (housing, nutrition, adult day care, and homemaker/chore services) to promote economic self-support and personal self-sufficiency for individuals with disabilities. Also, in 1974 the Developmental Disability Assistance and Bill of Rights Act also was passed. This legislation provides individuals with developmental disabilities the right to treatment, service, and habilitation and mandated University Affiliated Facilities to provide clinical service, manpower training, technical assistance on state of the art practice, and disseminate information on state of the art research findings and resources. This legislation, which includes social workers as one of the mandated professions to provide services, has benefited all individuals with disabling conditions.

Since the deinstitutionalisation movement began, the changes in the service and support system for individuals with developmental disabilities and their families have been dramatic. The University Affiliated Facilities established in the 1960s (now called University Affiliated Programmes) are situated in every state in the union and Puerto Rico. This network of University Affiliated Programmes provides manpower training for professionals from a wide range of disciplines who serve individuals with disabilities. These programmes also provide extensive interdisciplinary support and technical assistance to families, individuals with developmental disabilities, service providers, administrators, legislators and policymakers. The University Affiliated Programmes plan, develop and evaluate exemplary service programmes and support programmes, and they conduct research on developmental disabilities and human development. In addition many of these programmes have developed technological innovations, including assistive and adaptive computer technologies, to expand the motor and communication capabilities of individuals with disabling conditions (Vanderheiden & Dolan, 1985). Social workers have been an integral part of the development of the University Affiliated Programme network.

During the past two decades, the advocacy efforts of individuals with disabilities and their families, together with enlightened professionals representing a vast array of disciplines, have steadily led to the gradual acceptance of the rights of individuals with disabilities to determine the course of their lives as contributing members of the community and as citizens of a democratic society. Today the momentum is toward full inclusion of individuals with disabilities in all the cultural, social, economic and political aspects of community life. The passage of such legislation as:

- The Technology-Related Assistance Act which provides access to assistive technology services and devices for individuals with disabilities of all ages (1988);
- The Individuals with Disabilities Education Act which guarantees a free and appropriate education in the least-restrictive environment and supports interdisciplinary health and education services for children aged birth through 21 with disabling conditions and children at risk for disabling conditions (1990);
- The Americans with Disabilities Act which guarantees basic civil rights for all individuals with disabling conditions (1990); and
- The Rehabilitation Act which empowers individuals with disabilities from diverse racial/ethnic backgrounds to maximise employment, economic self-sufficiency, independence, and inclusion and integration into society (amended 1992).

These legislative enactments have established a framework that promotes the rights of individuals with disabilities as full citizens and support their inclusive participation in everyday community life.

The Role of Social Work from 1970 to the Present. In the 1970s, many individual social workers, and the profession as a whole, became more assertive, more independent, and played a key advocacy role in the movement toward deinstitutionalisation. As the emphasis shifted from institutional living to community integration and as the rights of the individual to choose his or her own

Social Work Practice Among Individuals with Disabling Conditions:
An Evolutionary Perspective

lifestyle in the community were endorsed, the service needs of individuals with disabilities have become increasingly complex and interwoven. This complexity often required the expertise of a constellation of professional disciplines. Today, interdisciplinary teams, working together with the individual who has a disability and his or her support system (family, friends and community caregivers), have become the accepted mode of practice. Social workers are recognised as important contributors and members of the interdisciplinary team whether they function in hospitals and clinics or in community-based programmes.

Fundamental to the practice of social work is the use of role theory and the commitment of social workers to using social roles to facilitate the involvement of an individual with a disability in their community. Social workers recognise that an individual with a disability is more than a patient or client and work to assist the individual to fulfil such varied social roles as family member, friend, employee, grocery shopper, transportation user, or participant in sports and leisure activities. Social workers foster a therapeutic climate which permits an individual with a disability to pursue and master diverse social roles.

In addition, social workers help to identify family and community resources and help to provide needed assistance and support. Disciplinary training in developmental theory, which articulates social role expectations at specific points in the lifespan, and training which underscores the social roles related to community life, strategically prepare social workers to make substantial contributions to the deliberations of interdisciplinary teams that serve individuals with disabilities.

Today, the role of social worker as liaison between families, the community, and the service sector continues to be an important social work function. Since the 1970s, however, the roles and functions of social workers have continued to broaden and expand. Today social workers serving individuals with disabilities are expected to have a working knowledge of:

- the systems (organisational and financial structures) within which services and supports are provided;
- the legislation and policies that shape service and support systems; and
- the social, cultural and demographic forces that bear upon the health and quality of life of individuals with disabilities.

Social workers are required to have the attributes, knowledge and skills needed to function as part of an interdisciplinary team, to provide direct services and supports for individuals with disabilities and their families, and to effect positive systems change at the community, state and national levels. The creation of new types of services such as group homes, supervised apartment living and special vocational-assistance programmes all require the community development and planning skills of social workers.

Social Work in the Twenty-First Century

As the social work profession faces the twenty-first century, numerous challenges must be addressed. In many ways these challenges result from the achievements of social workers as advocates for change throughout the twentieth century. As we move into the next century, social workers will most likely play a critical role in the movement toward independence, productivity, community integration, and the full inclusion of individuals with disabilities in all strands of society. Of particular importance will be the role of social workers as advocates, working together with families and individuals with disabilities to promote social change.

The struggle for true equality for persons with developmental disabilities will continue far into the twenty-first century. Within many communities, individuals are still shackled and limited by the historical social perspectives of individuals with disabilities as deviants and/or burdens on society. Social workers, along with other professionals who espouse full inclusion in society for individuals with disabilities, must often struggle against social strategies that promote paternalism and limit individual choice and freedoms.

As we move into the future, there is a growing demand among parents and other family members for a significant role in the formulation of public policy and in the planning, development, implementation, and evaluation of programme and service delivery systems for their children or relatives with disabilities. Many family members, particularly the parents of young children, are no longer willing to engage in the traditional and paternalistic methods used by many professionals who serve individuals with disabilities.

At times, there appears to be a growing antagonism between parents and professionals. Strategies must be identified and implemented to forge creative partnerships between parents and professionals. Both parents and professionals must work together to search for new ways to merge the technical expertise of professionals with the valid and relevant life experiences of parents and other family members. Family members and professionals have the potential to be formidable allies in the movement toward full inclusion and equality for all individuals with disabilities. As indicated earlier in this chapter, social workers have always played a major role in linking family members with the community

*Social Work Practice Among Individuals with Disabling Conditions:
An Evolutionary Perspective*

and the service system. Social workers are likely to be the most knowledgeable and skilled professionals to facilitate coalitions and alliances between family members and professionals to address the challenges of the twenty-first century.

Increasingly, advocates who themselves have disabilities are assuming leadership roles in setting the agenda for the pursuit of equality for individuals with disabilities. In the United States, this newly identified and invigorated leadership structure represents a social and civil rights movement that is growing in sophistication. However, the history of the movement toward full equality for individuals with disabilities is one which is, ironically, exclusionary.

It is increasingly evident that professionals, advocacy leaders, governmental officials, family members, and individuals with disabilities who are members of racial and ethnic minority groups are not a visible presence in the disability movement. While there is a disproportionate higher representation of racial and ethnic minority groups among individuals with disabilities, the leadership of the disability movement has remained almost totally composed of Americans of European descent. Such exclusionary policies have significantly reduced the credibility of the disability movement as a true movement for social and economic equality.

Beyond the reality of disability is the overarching reality of race, ethnicity and culture. Historically, individuals with disabilities from racial/ethnic minority groups have been doubly victimised — first, because of their primary identity as members of racial/ethnic minority groups which have been subject to racial discrimination and prejudice throughout the history of the country, and second, because of their disabilities (Kuehn & McClain, 1994). In the context of the global village that the world has become, this lack of diversity among the leadership in the disability movement represents a serious and tragic vestige of the past which must be addressed.

Social work advocacy must include campaigning for a serious and sustained recognition of the fundamental relationship between disability and culture. Racism and other discriminatory prejudices must be confronted directly if the disability movement is to succeed. The culture of disability itself is composed of many diverse cultures (racial, ethnic, religious, and geographic). In a democratic society, each of these cultures has an equal right to participate in the establishment of the national agenda for individuals with disabilities.

Social workers have an historical understanding of human relations and an ability to forge coalitions based on a recognition of common ground. The social workers in the twenty-first century should play a major role in facilitating culturally inclusive partnerships among individuals with disabilities, family members, and the professionals who provide education, health, rehabilitation, vocational, and social services for individuals with disabilities. Such partnerships at the community and national levels will be a critical force for designing a seamless advocacy, support and service system which is culturally diverse and able to support full citizenship for all people with disabilities.

The role and status of citizens in a democratic society bestow the right to a quality of life that is available to others and contributes to a sense of self which makes life worth living. A professional social worker's commitment is to creating that role and that quality of life for all members of society, including those who may be disadvantaged due to discrimination based on having a disabling condition.

References

Adams, M. (1971). *Mental retardation and its social dimensions.* NY: Columbia University Press.

Featherstone, H. (1981). *A difference in the family: Living with a disabled child.* NY: Penguin Books.

Horejsi, C. R. (1983). 'Developmental disabilities: Opportunities for social workers'; in *Developmental disabilities: No longer a private tragedy* (Ed. Lynn Wikler and Maryanne P. Keenan). Washington, DC: National Association of Social Workers, Inc.

Kuehn, M. and McClain, J. (1994). 'Quality of life: A multicultural context' in *Quality of life for people with disabilities: International perspectives and Issues.* (Ed. David A. Goode). Cambridge, Mass: Brookline Books.

Nacman, M. (1977). 'Social work in health settings: A historical review,' *Social Work in Health Care*; Vol. 2, No. 4.

Vanderheiden, G. and Dolan, T. (1985). 'Promises and concerns of technological intervention for children with disabilities' in *Developmental handicaps: Prevention and treatment.* Silver Spring, MD: American Association for University Affiliated Programmes.

Wikler, L. and Berkowitz, N. (1983). 'Social work, social problems and the mentally retarded' in *Developmental disabilities: No longer a private tragedy.* (Ed. L. Wikler and M. Keenan). Silver Spring, MD: National Association of Social Workers and Washington, DC: American Association on Mental Deficiency.

Wolfensberger, W. (1972). *The principle of normalisation in human services.* Toronto: National Institute on Mental Retardation.

Chapter 11
The Empowerment Framework: Bridging the Gap Between Individuals and Social Structures in Health Care

Audrey Mullender

Health can be thought of purely as the absence of illness or, more broadly, as a positive state of well-being. Seeing it as the former makes it the province of doctors and other health care professionals. The broader concept of well-being, however, only makes sense if individuals begin to take responsibility for their own health and to think of it in a holistic way — as affecting every aspect of daily life and the way they choose, or find themselves permitted, to live it.

A holistic concept of health encompasses the whole person: physical, mental, intellectual, emotional and spiritual elements of a whole being. The health care system has made a specialism of treating the body, the physical self. To a lesser extent, it has also staked a claim to expertise over mental functioning, by conceptualising it as a province of health or illness. Social work has traditionally been better then medicine at considering people in their entirety and in the context of their family, community and society. Social workers therefore have a major contribution to make to thinking about health. Furthermore, social work has been involved, in recent years, in developing ways of engaging people in taking responsibility for their own lives and for engendering change which could play an important role in fostering good health and improving health care.

A Model of Empowerment
In order to broaden our view of health to include our whole selves, we need to take back some of the control over deciding when we are well or ill, over ways of keeping well, and over our quality of life even when we do have an illness or a disability: in other words, we need a model of empowerment. The approach to empowerment which will be adopted for this chapter is based on that developed by Mullender and Ward (1991a and 1991b; Ward and Mullender, 1991). It is built on six principles which will be explored in the body of this chapter in terms of their relevance for thinking about health. Some examples will then explore the process of rethinking which occurs when those principles are followed in policy and practice (see Mullender and Ward, 1991b, for a more detailed account of empowering practice).

Principles for Empowerment
Principle 1
Social workers need to take a more rounded view of the people they work with, refusing to accept negative labels and recognising instead that all people have skills, understanding and ability.

The people with whom social workers engage must not be wrapped up or dismissed by the use of depersonalising generic terms such as 'the handicapped', or 'the sick'. One disabling characteristic which is labelled, or one illness condition which takes over a person's identity, can be enough to suck an individual into a system of treatment or containment, after which their whole functioning may be called into question and all opportunity for them to control their own lives removed. Once they are in the health care system, they are referred to as patients rather than people and their strengths, rights and individual characteristics become submerged.

Conditions which lead to this happening vary from country to country and from era to era. In Britain, there are still women alive who were placed for life in mental institutions because they had illegitimate babies and were considered to be morally defective. Even today, there are people in long-term institutional care because they have learning difficulties (formerly called mental handicaps), often combined with behaviour which others find hard to tolerate or manage, although they are increasingly moving to live in smaller hostels or group homes. Physical ill health now only leads to long-term hospitalisation if constant nursing care is required. Even then, there is a growing move towards providing this at home, as in kidney dialysis, or in a smaller and more personal setting where the whole person's spiritual and emotional needs, as well as their individual choices and qualities, can be noticed, such as in the hospice movement for terminally ill people. It would be unheard of in the West for someone to live in an institution because they have epilepsy, for example. This would be treated on a primary health care or out-patient basis. The differences which exist in national ways of responding to different levels of physical, mental or intellectual functioning depend largely on which conditions the health care system has traditionally exercised most power over, what decisions it has historically made about people 'suffering' from those conditions, and whether there have been others who have argued for increased rights to a normal life for that particular group.

Social workers have been closely involved in the movement out of the large institutions into a more integrated life in the community, where individuals previously written off as disabled or sick may exercise choices and rights on an equal basis

The Empowerment Framework: Bridging the Gap Between Individuals and Social Structures in Health Care

with other citizens. Social workers have seen that, not only do negative illness labels obscure the person, they also hide from view their strengths, skills, understanding, the ability to do things for themselves, and what they have to offer others. These strengths can most easily be tapped through shared endeavours in groups, including small-group living arrangements. Positive qualities are frequently underestimated, overlooked or disbelieved by people who fail to look beyond the labels imposed by health or other 'authorities'. Once people are accorded basic respect and seen again as people, however, they can emerge as retaining large areas of ability, of wellness, that had been forgotten by others and often by themselves.

This is one of the major revelations which social workers can offer through an empowering style of practice — they can help people to discover how strong, capable and aware they are, whatever their health care record, and to demonstrate what they can achieve for themselves. It is like going through the looking glass and finding that a world of quite different possibilities opens up on the other side. 'Humans are naturally powerful. The manifestations of powerlessness are only the social teachings we have digested' (Pike, undated, p.16). Traditionally, medicine has taught its patients powerlessness; it is for social work to teach them powerfulness.

When professionals new to the empowerment approach hear what members of groups have achieved — that they have set up self-advocacy representation across every geographical sector of a mental health service, for example, or obtained funding for a women's health centre and employed their own staff, or spoken at an international conference on disability — there is a fairly stock response of 'Oh, the people *I* work with could never do that'. Every health care professional who remains to be convinced resorts to the 'my patients are sicker than yours' line, which is another way of saying that his or her patients' views need not be listened to.

Yet sick and well people do break out of categories to which they have been assigned, either through their own efforts alone or because they begin to be listened to and encouraged to act on their own suggestions - including by social workers who see them in a fresh light. A wide range of groups of people, including users of mental health services, disabled people and people with learning difficulties, have benefited from their social workers' willingness to refuse to dismiss them with a negative and all-inclusive label but, instead, to see them as people with enormous potential.

Principle 2
People have rights, including the right to be heard and the right to control their own lives. It follows that people also have the right to choose what kinds of intervention and treatment to accept in their lives.

Once people's strengths and abilities are recognised, the social and health care which flows from this recognition has to accord people a far greater role in choosing what kinds of treatment and intervention they will accept in their lives, on the basis of full information about the alternatives.

Empowerment also means people finding their own voice. In the UK and the USA, for example, we have now become accustomed to hearing previously disempowered people appearing on national television and radio talking about their illnesses or disabilities and how they have fought back to retain dignity and control. They also, as representatives of local groups, address conferences and lead teaching sessions at in-service workshops and on professional training courses. Typically, these are people who have never been listened to before but, when they discover that their views are valued and can inspire others, they begin to find the words to express trenchant opinions and to describe negative experiences of limited lives or unacceptably poor treatment which should no longer be tolerated. Once people become more articulate, more confident, and more aware of their rights to good health, they may join with others to start a process of change either in the health care system itself or in relation to other aspects of life which have an adverse impact on health such as industrial pollution, tolerance of violence in the home, or harmful foods or drugs.

Principle 3
The range of factors that have an impact on people's health is complex; both organised health care and more informal responses need to reflect this. Health can never be fully understood if it is regarded solely as an issue of individual sickness or frailty. Issues of social policy, the environment and the economy are major contributory forces to ill health and need to be tackled in any movement towards improving the population's health.

Once patients' sickness labels begin to be challenged, and once their own views begin to be heard, it becomes more and more apparent that a complex range of factors in the health care and wider social system must change if a holistic perspective on health is to be pursued. Health and social work professionals may be daunted by this kind of analysis because they do not immediately see what relationship it can bear to their own everyday practice. Similarly, the general public may

The Empowerment Framework: Bridging the Gap Between Individuals and Social Structures in Health Care

feel that moving outside the privacy of the doctor:patient relationship is beyond their scope and not worth attempting.

Yet some of the biggest health advances in history have been made not by doctors but by public health measures with quite humble beginnings. The provision of clean water in a village or town, for example, can save many lives. In different parts of the world, citizens may take action for themselves to dig a new well, or they may direct their action towards demanding a new government which is more efficient at purifying the water supply. In eastern Europe, people are increasingly recognising that the drive towards centrally planned economic success was pursued with little or no regard to the risks of industrial pollution, including all manner of toxic discharges into the air and water or dangers of nuclear accident. These issues will only be taken more seriously if people insist that this must happen. There are many other ways in which ordinary people can take action to prevent death and disease. Research findings on preventative approaches — the linking of smoking with lung cancer, of excess alcohol with cirrhosis of the liver, of too much fat in the diet with many disorders including heart disease — of course have implications for individual changes in consumption of these products: the individual has to take responsibility for altering his or her diet or smoking or drinking habits. But they also have wider ramifications. Prevention requires official action in publicising the findings from research, in limiting the advertising of harmful products such as cigarettes or banning smoking in enclosed public places like the underground railway system (as has happened in London), or raising the price of harmful products through the imposition of taxes that lead people to cut down their use. It also requires a free press which takes seriously matters of social well-being and is prepared to report negligence and demand change. Ordinary people who care about their nation's health can demand such action and this can start at the local level, with professional support. For example a group of parents in England, whose children had been inhaling solvents (a popular form of substance misuse amongst young teenagers with no access to, or money for, drugs), got together to collect signatures on a petition demanding restrictions on the sale of solvents to unaccompanied young people and presented it to their Member of Parliament. They also held a meeting with local shopkeepers which led to voluntary changes in their town and attracted widespread coverage in the local media: radio, television and newspapers.

Regional or national differences in the provision of good health care are a matter of local and national concern. In Russia, the decreasing life expectancy, falling birthrate, high number of abortions and lack of access to other means of contraception (Ryan, 1994) have a complex range of causes including demographic change, economic circumstances requiring a national and international response, individual aspirations and economic activity amongst women, and male-dominated lifestyles and health agendas. But they can also be influenced by levels of awareness and assertiveness amongst women, and acceptance of responsibility by men, to demand change. The choice to limit births already shows women controlling their own destinies, even if the reasons are sometimes forced on them by hardship. It is a shorter step from there to demanding healthier options than they have already taken to reach this point. Similarly, the health care system alone cannot cope with epidemic cardiovascular disease or alcohol misuse (Schultz and Rafferty, 1990) but will depend on major change ranging from individual choices in diet and leisure to social policies governing the well-being of the nation.

This is where the practice of empowerment, and not just its principles, comes into play. The view that wider social problems can begin to be resolved through individual choice followed by campaigning at a localised level, when people come together in groups to pursue their own goals for change, has led to many doors which have appeared shut in the past beginning to open. Typically, an unbridgeable gap has been assumed to exist between what the individual practitioner or citizen can set in motion on the one hand and the sort of changes which would require government instigation or some other form of official action on the other. People who are accustomed to waiting for macro-level activity feel powerless. This leads us directly onto the fourth principle.

Principle 4
People acting together can be powerful; people who lack power can gain it through working together in groups.

What needs to happen, then, is to draw people together into groups to empower them to tackle problems external to themselves, normally on a localised basis at first, but often broadening out to attain regional or national dimensions when tackled in conjunction with others. Any aspect of health care can be improved through group-based efforts based on local people knowing what needs to change and taking action to make or demand that change. Examples can range from a group of parents of children with asthma raising funds for equipment in local surgeries to prevent their children being hospitalised during acute attacks (Wilson, 1986: 130), to people with HIV/AIDS setting up a telephone helpline. A group of women who were committed to the idea of being able to choose where to give birth (Wilson, 1986: 129), used evidence that many deliveries are as safe at home as in hospital to focus its efforts on making both available options.

The Empowerment Framework: Bridging the Gap Between Individuals and Social Structures in Health Care

Through groups of individuals such as these, often the wider communities of interest which they represent are also empowered. This may consist of the broader group of people with the same illness or disability, the same industrial disease, or the same suffering as a result of medical or pharmaceutical negligence. There are not only local groups but national campaigning organisations in Britain associated with asthma, AIDS and childbirth, for example.

Social workers may assist this process of bringing people together who share similar experiences so that their professional intervention is directed explicitly at helping those who are relatively powerless to aquire more power. To help in this way, social and health care professionals must be willing really to hear when service users say that structural problems are having an impact on their lives, rather than resorting to the old labels of sickness or inadequacy. They must not be tempted to refashion the problem into something individual which can be seen as more amenable to expert 'packaging' of sickness into neat pigeon-holes. There are important messages here for practitioners which are reflected in the next principle.

Principle 5
Professionals do not 'lead' but facilitate people in making decisions for themselves and in controlling whatever outcome ensues. Though special skills and knowledge are employed, these do not accord privilege and are not solely the province of the professionals.

Workers must want to work *with* people and not to direct intervention *to* or *at* them. The professional must consequently be a facilitator rather than a leader or expert in the traditional sense, which has quite different power connotations. Power is never value-free or value-neutral and leadership can never be simply a technical exercise in management; it necessarily stems from explicit or implicit intentions and purposes which, if left to default, will reinforce rather than question dominant social values. Empowerment relies on asking who determines those intentions and purposes as a pre-requisite of handing back the power over decision-making to the wider public.

Just as the professional may need time to develop a new role and fresh skills, so the public they serve, too, may need time to become accustomed to looking to each other rather than to the experts for answers. People are more used to professionals as authority figures, and as resource providers. Consequently, they may expect to be told what to do and how to do it; it takes practice in working together for group members to recognise that they can look to the professionals for help but not for instruction. The refusal to be directive, without falling into being totally non-directive, can be difficult, but the process is necessary if ordinary people are to take responsibility for their own groups and for their own health care campaigns.

The professional's firm placing of responsibility back with the emerging group may have to continue, intermittently, throughout a group's life; for example, one women's health group had been in existence for several years and had moved on to employing its own worker, but she still found that the group occasionally attempted to pass decision-making to her; she then needed to remind members of how much they had achieved already, and to stress that new tasks and responsibilities were not beyond their capabilities. In ways such as this, it can be appropriate for workers to be directive in relation to *process* in order to ensure that they are never directive in relation to *goals*.

Social workers can assist with finding ways to achieve a group's desired ends, then, but should not dictate what those ends will be. This style of working is essential if the earlier principles are to be observed. Opening themselves up to hearing what service users are saying (Principle 2), empowering them to set their own goals (Principle 3), and taking shared action (Principle 4), imply drawing out the best from group members and helping them to determine where they want the group to go, rather than imposing other agendas on them.

There is certainly no less skill involved in this kind of work than in groupwork which is led from the centre. Groups can require facilitation at any or all stages of the process: in coming together to share their experiences, in finding the means to form views and set goals, and in generating the knowledge and skills needed to carry out tasks.

Principle 6
Social work must challenge all forms of oppression, whether by reason of race, gender, sexual orientation, age, class, disability, or any other form of social differentiation upon which spurious notions of superiority and inferiority are developed and kept in place by the exercise of power.

All nations, at different points in time, regard certain sections of their population as inherently inferior. This has happened to people of Romany origin and of the Islamic faith in eastern Europe, and to people of African, Asian and Hispanic origin in western Europe and north America, as well as to guestworkers, refugees and immigrants moving to seek safety, shelter or sustenance in many parts of the world. Virtually all over the globe, too, men have misused their greater physical strength and their ability to neglect child-rearing roles to devote themselves to

The Empowerment Framework: Bridging the Gap Between Individuals and Social Structures in Health Care

monopolising power and control in all domains of policy formulation and enactment. Social background, age, sexuality, and levels of real or supposed physical wholeness or wellness have been used to create social hierarchies in similar ways. The Nazi concentration camps brought together all these abominations in holding mentally ill and disabled people, including those with learning difficulties, as well as Jewish, Romany and gay people, while young fit women of Aryan stock were required to devote themselves to producing children for the Fatherland.

Social workers need to understand and oppose all these forms of oppression through their work. Until homophobia is tackled, for example, there will continue to be obstacles to providing good health care for one of the groups most at risk of HIV infection. It is not enough to think about forms of oppression individually, however; to be anti-racist or anti-sexist, to tackle issues of disability or of age, class or sexuality. Empowerment requires an analysis which conceptualises the processes of oppression as interlinked, their impact as overlapping (for a black disabled woman, for example), and the processes of change as needing to move forward on all fronts at once.

Groups often find this difficult to achieve in practice, even those projects which have gone a very long way with the other five principles and whose whole driving force is to combat negative treatment of their particular interest group within society. They still may have considerably further to go in pursuing the principle of general anti-oppressive working, and in seeing the various forms of oppression as interlinked. Thus it is not uncommon, when groups of disabled people or ex-psychiatric patients first start, for example, for them to be more successful initially in empowering their white male members to speak out and to take committee positions. Special efforts are often required to develop an equal opportunities policy for the organisation, and to debate the issues so that white male participants recognise that the group cannot speak for its entire constituency until it gives an equal voice and equal representation to black people and women, and to people with a range of disabilities or recovering from a range of mental illness diagnoses. Social workers can have a facilitative role in fostering this broader view of oppressive processes in groups they advise or support.

These, then, are the six principles underpinning an empowering model of social work. This chapter will now turn to two examples of service user groups whose view of the world has completely changed because these principles have been followed. They are women with mental health problems and disabled people. Both were formerly accustomed to having their lives controlled and their choices dictated by medical decisions, to which social workers were also subservient. The challenge to social work is now to accept — and indeed to harness its skills to fostering — the viewpoint which the empowerment of women and of disabled people has achieved.

The specific focus in this chapter on women's mental health is not intended to imply either that men do not suffer from mental illnesses or that the stress of modern living does not take its particular toll of men's health and wholeness. A society in which men have severe constraints placed upon their choices and freedom of movement, where they must play a rigidly socially defined role of aggressive masculinity, and yet which leaves them unable to provide for their families in the way they have been brought up to believe is their duty, is likely to create considerable emotional and mental stress which may manifest itself in alcohol or drug misuse, or in mental ill health. These issues need attention alongside other aspects of a rapidly changing world which is looking for a new order for all humanity. Nevertheless, it is valid to focus on women's particular mental health needs for three reasons. First, women face constraints, rigidities and abuses caused by their prescribed social role in most countries of the world. Second, they face these limitations and injustices over and above those endured by their wider community in relation, for example, to poverty or political repression. Third, this fact has begun to be recognised and has led in consequence to a careful analysis of the nature of women's oppression and of possible empowering responses to it which can not only bring new hope to women but also offer lessons for all people who feel oppressed by their circumstances. It is not necessary to be female and/or disabled to be enriched by the experiences and insights outlined below.

Examples of Rethinking Health Issues
through the Empowerment of Health Care Recipients
Women and Mental Health
Recent years have seen an increasing awareness in the West that mainstream psychiatric services do not provide the most appropriate response to women's mental health needs. Women themselves have voiced their discontent and rejected the traditional labels and inadequate treatment. In the UK, for example, a number of campaigns and publications have raised questions (Barnes and Maple, 1992; MIND, 1992; MIND 1994), including why the typical response to women should have to veer between neglect and over-treatment (Community Care, 19-25 May 1994: 14). The efforts to achieve change build on a tradition in sociology (Brown *et al.*, 1975; Brown and Harris, 1978; Miles, 1988) and social work (Corob, 1987), of trying to reach an understanding of how mental ill health — notably depression —

The Empowerment Framework: Bridging the Gap Between Individuals and Social Structures in Health Care

affects women and drawing out some of the reasons in relation to family responsibilities, social isolation and female social roles. As early as 1972, Gove (1972) had demonstrated that marriage is good for men's mental health and bad for women's. What are seen as 'normal' social expectations can actually make women sick.

The revelation of sexism within the psychiatric system has also clarified our thinking and is, again, far from new. Broverman *et al.* (1970) showed mental health professionals exhibiting sex bias: in an experiment, clinicians attributed similar characteristics to a 'mature, healthy, socially competent' man as to an adult with sex unspecified, but they chose quite different words from a given list to describe a healthy woman. The greater emphasis on passivity, dependency, submissiveness, being emotional and excitable, and so on, that they expected to see in normal, healthy women showed both that the professionals' notion of an 'adult' equated with a man and that they were operating double standards in their definitions of good health. These could certainly lead to the misdiagnosis of women who failed to accord with the biased 'norms'. This can happen very easily in any society where women are not accorded equal respect with men. Recent criticisms of the psychiatric system have grown still more trenchant in revealing, for example, sexual harassment and sexual violence in psychiatric settings, not only by therapists (Teevan, 1991) but also by other patients in mixed institutions (MIND, 1992).

There is a growing movement towards women finding their own solutions outside mainstream services (Women in MIND, 1986), chiefly through women-only groups facilitated by other women who use an empowering process in their work. At the Women's Therapy Centre in London, for example (Ernst and Goodison, 1981; Krzowski and Land, 1988), workshops have covered issues such as agoraphobia or depression, as well as groups aimed specifically at black women, working-class women and lesbian women, and groups to develop creativity or body-awareness. Other women find healing and raised awareness in therapy, groupwork, or community activity of various kinds in their local communities. All in all, women's groups, workshops and campaigns keep many women well — or at least out of the hands of the psychiatric services where their needs are often poorly understood and the treatments and attitudes they encounter tend to make them feel worse rather than better.

Recently, an initiative was taken by the European Regional Council of the World Federation for Mental Health to identify and develop good practice in mental health services for women. The results of the UK element of this work have included an information pack (Good Practices in Mental Health [GPMH], 1994) and a training pack (Andrews *et al.*, 1994). Although the former aims 'to make visible and celebrate the good work which is already being done' it is also clear about the need to provide inspiration and guidance to those who want to fill the gaps' (GPMH, 1994, Introduction, p.2). The packs both stress that women use mental health services more than men. In England, 58 per cent of all psychiatric admissions are women (Health and Personal Social Services Statistics for England, 1987, HMSO, cited in Andrews *et al.*, 1994) and women also consult primary health care services more frequently on grounds of mental or emotional distress. Yet women do not consider that their needs are met by existing health care. This starts with the most basic issues of service provision, such as a lack of mother and baby units in psychiatric hospitals and of crèche facilities in day hospitals. it also includes the therapeutic issues of inappropriate treatments and the lack of an analysis of mental distress which takes account of causative experiences such as sexual abuse in childhood or violence and other abuse from adult partners.

Amongst the largest groups of women using psychiatric services are survivors of child sexual abuse and of physical and/or sexual abuse in adult relationships, yet traditional diagnostic techniques do not engage with these wider social issues. Work in the USA (Jacobson *et al.*, 1987; Jacobson and Richardson, 1987, cited in Andrews *et al.*, 1994) found that, compared with self-report, 100 sets of psychiatric case-notes missed 100 per cent of both childhood and adult sexual assaults, as well as 85 per cent of childhood and 90 per cent of adult physical assaults. Whilst not denying the real depression and anxiety that these experiences can cause, it does seem an indictment that a major response of contemporary society is to blame the victim by labelling her as sad or mad and offering treatments which do nothing to help raise her awareness of the abuse as not her fault.

Women are beginning to be empowered to voice their own demands for better mental health care and for a less 'sick' society which will devote more energy and resources to helping them keep well. A more positive response to women's mental, emotional and spiritual health, needs to take into account that women are not one homogeneous group. Ethnic diversity, disability, financial hardship, age, marital status and sexual orientation can all create particular needs — and particular strengths to offer to other women. A different perspective will be held by a women in urban and in rural areas, by young women, women who are carers of dependent relatives, or women identified as offenders, as well as those who misuse alcohol or drugs or are addicted to prescription medicines such as tranquillisers. Women may also have child-related needs which include post-natal depression and reactions to losing a child (GPMH, 1994). There is a wide-ranging need for change. At present, older women are prescribed more drugs despite greater risk of side effects, health professionals commonly still see lesbian sexuality as a cause of mental health problems, and racist services affect black women adversely, for example through the lack of black counsellors (Andrews *et al.*, 1994). Members of each of these groups of women can come together to take action on their own account and mixed groups of women need to be aware of this broad range of concerns.

Two social workers helped to set up a 'women and health' group in an area of public-owned housing where poverty and unemployment were high and poor health and depression were common. Their first problem was to encourage women out of their homes to attend a meeting. A community centre on the estate was used for an informal chat over coffee and, as many of the women were single parents, a crèche was provided. Starting from this informal social gathering, the women agreed that they wanted to meet again and they brought others along. They began to discuss health-related issues and stress-inducing problems related to cuts in jobs and child-care provision. With support from the group-workers, women from 25 to 70 years of age raised funds to set up children's playschemes and after-school clubs; they also encouraged each other to gain qualifications, initially by inviting tutors in to run courses in the community centre until they felt confident enough to go back to college. Some are now studying at local universities. Throughout this time, the women have run health-awareness days through which they have made the links between social conditions and women's mental health. Most recently, they have raised money with other local groups to visit the European Parliament to raise issues of preventive health care for women.

All mental health and social workers need to challenge accepted stereotypes and to promote better practice for women from a wide range of social backgrounds in their own workplace. This should include respecting the contribution of the women who work there. The key element is aiming at awareness-raising and confidence-building to help women exercise choice over their own lives.

Disability Redefined

Physically 'put away' over the years into institutional care, disabled people have also been pigeon-holed and dismissed by labels, assumptions and stereotypical responses as if they were infants, invalids or objects. These labels set disabled people apart, be they of the negative and depersonalising variety — 'cripples', 'the handicapped' — or the equally objectionable positive labels such as 'courageous', 'inspiring' and 'brave'. Both are sides of the same coin. Disability is conceptualised as a personal tragedy whether the individual is seen as being overwhelmed by it or as fighting back (Shearer, 1981, pp.20-23). Sometimes the imagery becomes confused as when a terminally ill child was shown on British television crying bitterly while being described as 'brave little James'. Oliver (1983, p.20) regards both sets of exaggerations as convenient in apparently letting social workers off the hook, since their efforts to help can be interpreted as either pointless or superfluous. A new generation of social workers are beginning to refuse to fall into that trap and are taking a lead from disabled people themselves in encouraging them to feel empowered to seek change.

Organisations of disabled people increasingly reject the concept of disability as a set of symptoms with consequent physical limitations necessitating psychological adjustment. Instead they choose to see disability as a *social phenomenon*. Indeed, they regard it as caused by a society which takes no account of people with physical impairments and thus excludes them from participation in the mainstream of social activities (UPIAS, 1976; Finkelstein, 1980, p.33). Taking this view, the goal a social worker should seek with a newly disabled person or with the parent of a disabled baby is not adjustment to a limited life-style or mourning for a loss but introduction to others who, by taking action and speaking out together, can press for better provision of services and an end to socially imposed limitations.

What is highlighted here is a structural, not an individual, set of circumstances which can be addressed by groups of disabled people working together to achieve change. The choice for social workers becomes whether to support the effort for change or whether to impede it, if only by apathy and default. Increasingly, social workers are offering more than moral support by becoming active allies in establishing and supporting the groups which are seeking change.

They are providing backing for groups and organisations of disabled people who are no longer content to be a low priority group, required to satisfy stringent eligibility criteria and join long waiting-lists for essential services. Nor are disabled people content to be counselled into 'coming to terms' with their 'problems'. Rather their organisations are demanding practical solutions to practical problems such as dressing, using the toilet, and cooking. 'What I need is someone who will help me to achieve these things with as little fuss as possible, allowing me to preserve my personal integrity at the same time' (Vernon, 1986, p.28).

Social work help traditionally was not offered on these terms. It came with an accompaniment of psychological assumptions focusing on adjustment to loss. Believing that we, as helping professionals, have the right to define someone else as having suffered a fundamental loss is patronising. It regards the disabled person as lacking something basic which we have and they do not. It ignores the fact that, even without that function, they may still be a more whole or rounded person than us — more intelligent perhaps, more musical, or more fun to be with. The obvious question is whose concept of normality we choose to adopt. All are socially created and relative. They are also self-defined: 'you see to me the way I am is "normal"' (Sheila Roberts in Nicholls *et al.*, 1985, p.23).

Hence, the traditional social work emphasis on therapy for disabled people, to achieve adjustment, is often entirely misplaced. One of the stages of loss which social workers are taught must be overcome in this process of 'adjustment' is that of anger. Unacceptable attitudes and behaviour will never be changed unless disabled people stay angry and channel their anger into action for change. Perhaps it is for our own comfort that we expect them to become inured to limitations which are *not* inevitable and which we would not wish to accept for ourselves. Having this aim as part of an accepted theory makes it respectable but not, it is suggested, unchallengeable.

All too often, disabled people find that going to a traditionally orientated agency to seek essentially practical help makes them fair game to be turned into 'clients' by old style social workers, rather than simply being given the required assistance. The person who has gone along to enquire about housing, income or jobs, is made to feel that the social worker wants to dabble in his or her whole life, asking questions about feelings and relationships (Crine, 1982: 26), even if the disabled person considers these wholly irrelevant to the barrier or obstacle to daily living which he or she is trying to overcome. Being labelled as a 'client' can mean being expected to be a passive recipient of intrusive intervention and required to accept the 'expert's' definition of the problem.

Social workers, however unwittingly, become part of the fabric of the social oppression of disabled people when they accept a medical model which casts them into rigid roles as dependent or helpless clients whose sole responsibility is to adjust, unquestioningly, to a restricted life, 'learning to live with' obstacles to participation, 'coming to terms with' barriers to choice. As Oliver says, 'Adjustment . . . [should be] a problem for society, not for disabled individuals' (Oliver, 1983, p.23). How far is society willing to adjust its patterns and expectations to include its members who have disabilities and to remove handicaps that society itself imposes? Unless there is significant progress in this direction, it will not only be the individual who suffers. All disabled people are damaged, and indeed all of us are lessened, by a view of disability which limits the problem to the level of individual conformity and thereby conceals the discrimination caused by inadequate provision.

Disabled people are increasingly unwilling to be moved into segregated establishments. 'We . . . stopped going to day-centres as we didn't agree with them. We wanted to live life as normal as we possibly could' (John Roberts in Nicholls *et al.*, 1985, p.25, writing about himself and his wife, Sheila). In contrast, organisations run by disabled people, like the centres for integrated living in a number of British cities, offer a comprehensive service, encompassing advice and help with housing, transport, technical aids, environmental access, personal assistance with self-care, education and employment. They are able to help an individual design an appropriate package of services to meet his or her own needs and to co-ordinate these for someone wishing to live independently in the community, for example. Shearer (1981, p.179) regards this new style of campaigning as 'a challenge . . . to traditional concepts of charitable endeavour for people who are, by definition, to be 'done to', who are seen as helpless, pitiable'. Oliver (1983, p.24) characterises the key questions to be asked of professionals as 'whether they wish to work for disabled people or with them'. This involves an inevitable reconsideration of the distribution of power and influence between helper and helped (Finkelstein, 1980, p.13).

Disabled people, through their own organisations, are increasingly represented on committees determining health and welfare priorities and in policy-making exercises. An invitation to join such a forum may still be tokenistic, however, unless buildings are physically accessible to wheelchair users, committee papers are available in braille or in large print, and signed interpretation and induction loops are offered for deaf people and those who are hard of hearing. Furthermore, as people with learning difficulties also increasingly demand to take their rightful place as full citizens, social workers' whole concept of communication in meetings may need to shift so that, instead of hiding behind jargon (which often we could not fully explain if challenged), we will need to explain what we really mean, in straightforward language, and show that we mean it through concrete achievements. We will also have to give others adequate space to voice their demands and concerns (Advocacy in Action, 1989/90, p.4).

Full participation requires more than a letter of invitation to a meeting. It also requires a move away from tokenism. As with representation of women and black people, there can be a tendency in official circles to think that the demands of consultation and involvement have been fulfiled if just one disabled person is present:

The Empowerment Framework: Bridging the Gap Between Individuals and Social Structures in Health Care

So often you get committees, you get all these people who, I know it sounds dreadful, think they are doing so much good, but they never stop and think 'right, what do the disabled themselves think?' ... and then when you say something, they get really very hurt that you are criticising all their hard work ... but if only they would have stopped first and said 'let's consult the disabled' ... or what is just as insulting, like the statutory woman, have a disabled person on sufferance, but they don't really want to know what you think, they just want you there to make the numbers up and just be seen. (Muriel in Campling, 1981, p.117.)

We need to ask ourselves whether we do really want to know what disabled people think — including their views of us as social work professionals and the services we provide — or whether we would rather take the easy way out and find one of the many ploys to avoid hearing. Have we the strength to make the changes they will demand, however radical these may be and however they may strike at the heart of traditional residential and day care provision and time-honoured theories of loss, for example? If we have, then the empowerment model and its six principles show us how we can be involved as part of the solution to the needs of sick and disabled people, rather than part of the problem.

Conclusion

Our understanding of disability and ill health must resemble our understanding of any form of social oppression, to which we need to respond with empowering skills and ideas. Borrowing a link made some years ago by the women's movement, the *personal* experience of sickness or disability becomes a *political* understanding of social divisions. Groups of people with health-related problems are coming together to take control over their own lives, together with the collective power to question public and professional attitudes, to challenge societal prejudice and oppression, and to demand a socially integrated life. Many of these groups and organisations are keen to enter into a dialogue with their local social services about the most positive role for social workers and about a joint striving for more enlightened policies. The British Council of Organisations of Disabled People, for example, has sought to hold formal dialogues with social services departments as to how they can adapt to a new view of, and new demands being voiced by, disabled people. In Britain, too, empowering values and skills are now universally taught on social work qualifying courses which should mean that the social workers of the future will know how to welcome and work with the strengths in all those they work with and not their negative labels.

This move towards change will be empowering for workers as well as for service users. It removes the barriers imposed by traditions of 'therapy' or 'treatment' and enables us to find our common humanity with those with whom we work. It also means that, although we retain expertise as professional workers, we do not operate in a style which suggests we have all the answers. Obstacles and challenges encountered by the group as it proceeds towards its goals are shared with the group as a whole, to be discussed and resolved jointly. This typically leads to the discovery of solutions more in keeping with the overall direction the group has chosen, and more dependent on the combined strength of the group — thus serving at the same time to reaffirm the group's sense of identity and purpose.

It has not been the intention of this chapter to suggest that the empowerment model of practice is the approach of choice in every situation. There are times when an individual is simply too unwell, or too withdrawn, to participate in a group, or when this would not be their personal choice. There will always be a need for individual help and treatment to be available. Even then, however, there may well be a role for a collective voice of ordinary people — who have, or have had, similar problems — to help ensure that treatment standards are set and observed at a sufficiently high standard and that medical, social work and other staff are open to outside influence, not purely self-regulation. Some patients or users of social services who receive individual assistance will later wish to graduate to membership of such a 'watchdog' body, as happens with Community Health Councils in Britain, for example. It should be personal need and preference, not organisational rigidity or resource limitations, which determine people's access either to individualised services or to empowerment groups — and involvement in both at once is by no means uncommon. In this way, a community gets the level of service it demands and works to achieve through advocating on its own behalf.

References

Advocacy in Action/People for People Forum (1989/90) *Annual Report — Working Together,* Princes House, 32 Park Row, Nottingham NG1 6GR: Advocacy in Action /People for People Forum.

Andrews, C., Nadirshaw, Z., Curtis, Z. and Ellis, J. (1994) *Women, Mental Health and Good Practice,* Brighton: Pavilion Publishing.

Barnes, M. and Maple, N. (1992) *Women and Mental Health: Challenging the Stereotypes,* Birmingham: Venture Press.

Broverman, I., Broverman, D., Clarkson, F., Rosenkrantz, P. and Vogal, S. (1970) 'Sex-role stereotypes and clinical judgements of mental health', *Journal of Consulting and Clinical Psychology*, 34, 1-7.

Brown, G. W., Brochlain, M. and Harris, T. (1975) 'Social class and psychiatric disturbance among women in an urban population', *Sociology*, 9, 225-254.

Brown, G. W. and Harris, T. (1978) *Social Origins of Depression*, London: Tavistock.

Campling, J., ed. (1981) *Images of Ourselves: Women with Disabilities Talking*, London, Boston and Henley: Routledge and Kegan Paul.

Community Care (19-25 May 1994), pp.14-15, p.18 and p.21.

Corob, A. (1987) *Working with Depressed Women: A Feminist Approach*, Aldershot: Gower.

Crine, A. (1982) 'Was ever a battle like this?', *Community Care*, (422) 24-26.

Ernst, S. and Goodison, L. (1981) *In Our Own Hands: A Book of Self-Help Therapy*, London: The Women's Press.

Finkelstein, V. (1980) *Attitudes and Disabled People: Issues for Discussion* New York: World Rehabilitation Fund Inc. Reprinted by London: RADAR, Monograph no. 5.

Good Practices in Mental Health (1994) *Women and Mental Health: An Information Pack of Mental Health Services for Women in the United Kingdom*, London: GPMH (Publications Dept, 380-384 Harrow Road, London W9 2HU).

Gove, W. R. (1972) 'The relationship between sex roles, marital status and mental illness', *Social Forces*, 51(1), 34-44.

Jacobson, A., Koehler, J. E. and Jones-Brown, C. (1987) 'The failure of routine assessment to detect histories of assault experienced by psychiatric patients', *Hospital and Community Psychiatry,* 38(4), pp.386-389.

Jacobson, A. and Richardson, B. (1987) 'Assault experience of 100 psychiatric inpatients: evidence of need for routine inquiry', *American Journal of Psychiatry*, 144(7), pp.908-913.

Krzowski, S. and Land, P., eds (1988) *In Our Experience: Workshops at the Women's Therapy Centre*, London: The Women's Press.

Miles, A. (1988) *Women and Mental Illness: The Social Context of Female Neurosis*, Brighton: Wheatsheaf.

MIND (1992) *Stress on Women* London: MIND (pack).

MIND (1994) *Eve Fights Back: Report on MIND's 'Stress on Women' Campaign* London: MIND.

Mullender, A. and Ward, D. (1991a) *The Practice Principles of Self-Directed Groupwork: Establishing a Value-Base for Empowerment,* Nottingham: University of Nottingham, Centre for Social Action.

Mullender, A. and Ward, D. (1991b) *Self-Directed Groupwork: Users Take Action for Empowerment,* London, Whiting and Birch.

Nicholls, J., O'Hara, W., Trotman, A., Roberts, J. and S., Shaban, N., Young People from the Link Unit, Minihane, S., MacCallum, S., 1985, *A Celebration of Differences: A Book by Physically Handicapped People, 108c Stokes Croft,* Bristol BS1 3RU: Bristol Broadsides [Co-op] Ltd.

Oliver, M. (1983) *Social Work with Disabled People,* London: Macmillan.

Pike, E. (undated) *Empowerment; Personal and Political Change,* Philadelphia, PA, USA: Movement for a New Society.

Ryan, M. (1994) 'Mother Russia', in *Health Service Journal,* 26 May, 22-23.

Schultz, D. S. and Rafferty, M. P. (1990) 'Soviet health care and perestroika', *American Journal of Public Health,* 80(2), 193-197.

Shearer, A. (1981) *Disability: Whose Handicap?* Oxford: Basil Blackwell.

Teevan, S. (1991) *Women Who Are Abused by Their Therapists,* London: MIND.

Union of the Physically Impaired Against Segregation (1976) *Fundamental Principles of Disability* London: UPIAS and the Disability Alliance.

Vernon, G. (1986) 'Untrained carers are tops', *Community Care* (628) 11 September: 28-29.

Ward, D. and Mullender, A. (1991) 'Empowerment and oppression: an indissoluble pairing for contemporary social work', *Critical Social Policy,* 11(2), Issue 32, pp.21-30.

Wilson, J. (1986) *Self-Help Groups: Getting Started — Keeping Going,* Harlow: Longman.

Women in MIND (1986) *Finding Our Own Solutions: Women's Experience of Mental Health Care,* London: MIND.

Chapter 12
Preparing Social Workers for Practice in Health Care

Norma Berkowitz and Lowell Jenkins

This chapter (1) briefly reviews the concepts and themes stressed in this book, (2) presents what is known about the kinds of health settings in which professionally trained social workers are employed in the United States and the kinds of services they provide, (3) specifies some curriculum objectives, and (4) concludes with some reflections on challenges facing social workers concerned about the health status of people who are vulnerable because of health-related conditions or who are at serious risk for developing life-threatening conditions because of (a) severely limited economic resources devoted to health care systems, (b) limited access to health resources that do exist, or (c) are at the mercy of environmental policies that disregard health risks.

Review of Concepts and Themes
There are four major themes stressed throughout this book: (1) the social work profession's commitment to fostering a humane society and environment for those who are ill or have a disabling condition; (2) an approach to social work practice which facilitates a holistic perspective on human behaviour that includes the interaction of individuals and groups with biological, psychological, and social environments; (3) social work has both a social reform history that focused on promoting and safeguarding health and as well as a history of service to helping people already afflicted; (4) in regard to health, social work practice has a role in preventing illness, promoting and maintaining health as well as serving those who are already affected by illness or adverse health conditions.

Whether working as a public health, prevention-oriented social worker or as a social worker providing direct services to those who are already ill or disabled, the model of practice proposed as most suitable is that of the generalist. The components of this model are set out in chapter 1. Subsequent chapters illustrate the need for the multi-systems level assessments and interventions that are the central feature of generalist practice.

Social work process is presented in each chapter and the process emerges as having common characteristics:

(1) it is structured; (2) it is a mutual and shared process with other colleagues as well as with those being served and maximises the participation of those *receiving* help or assistance; (3) power is shared between those seeking assistance and those *providing* assistance; (4) it is goal directed, problem solving and behaviourally oriented.

Intervention processes were illustrated in each chapter. Several underlying themes emerged: (1) the *person environment focus* in social work practice; (2) the overwhelming importance of *multidisciplinary collaboration*; (3) the importance of *social support and coping* on the part of those suffering from illness or disability; (4) the use of *classification systems* which may result in positive or negative consequences; (5) social work's concern with both an *individual* and *collective* focus and both a social reform and a therapeutic mission.

For illustrative purposes the book presented four frameworks, or ways of viewing, social work practice:

(1) *The Systems' Framework* is the basic theory which underlies contemporary social work and is embedded in the world view which helps form problem identification and assess levels of potential intervention (individual, group, community, society). The systems framework is embedded in the bio-psychosocial framework in chapters 2, 3, 4; the public health framework in chapters 5, 6, 7; and the empowerment framework in chapters 10 and 11. Social work strategies developed to enhance access to, and utilisation of, services (chapters 8 and 9) also rest on a system perspective.

(2) *The Bio-Psychosocial Framework* stressed comparison of a 'medical model', disease-oriented approach to 'caring versus curing' and a holistic, humanistic approach to providing health care and services. The chapters on alcohol use (chapter 2) hospital social work (chapter 3), and palliative care (chapter 4) each addressed a social problem area from the standpoint of a holistic approach to health-related problems, emphasising that quality of life is an important aspect for people even when cure is not possible.

(3) *The Public Health Framework* is oriented to a social work tradition that focuses on the general welfare of at-risk and underserved populations. Within this framework lie the philosophy and the strategies which enable social work to focus on health promotion, maintenance of health status, and preventive interventions. The chapter on primary care (chapter 5) explores issues, advantages and possibilities of combining public health strategies with private medical group practices, a model for providing primary care which attempts to blend the curative and preventive aspects of providing care. For social work, the model attempts to clarify the generalist and the public health social work role in these settings. The chapter on family planning in Russia (chapter 6) identified the opportunity for utilising public health concepts to facilitate birth spacing, thereby maximising the potential for the health of mothers and children. The family planning chapter and the AIDS chapter (chapter 7) highlighted a social work specialist role dedicated to using

public health primary prevention strategies. The AIDS chapter also illustrated the in-depth knowledge about the human body and disease processes that the social worker must have in order to successfully work as a specialist with a population suffering from a complex medical condition.

(4) *The Empowerment Framework* was highlighted in the chapter on the historical process which moved those with disabling and handicapping conditions from the institution to the community (chapter 10) and the empowerment chapter on bridging the gap between individuals and social structures (chapter 11). However, in describing the social work process as it occurred in each chapter presentation, empowerment (formal or informal and of varying degrees) is a theme underlying all of the chapters. This framework directly and continually challenges social work practitioners to view their own stereotypes, their own attitudes about the place in society of those who are 'different', and the risks social workers are willing to undertake on behalf of the clients they serve. Although the two chapters on utilisation and access to services were highlighted in a separate section, work with refugees (chapter 8) and work in the community with those with severe mental illness (chapter 9) deal primarily with empowering people to live their lives in the community as unencumbered as possible by their difficulties.

Several *themes* also emerge: (1) the concept of *person:environment interactions* as the central focus for social work practice in health care; (2) the overwhelming importance of *multidisciplinary collaboration in the health care arena*; (3) social work's *commitment to both individuals and collectives*; (4) the need of those with health-related problems for *social support* throughout the illness trajectory and sometimes throughout the life-span.

A theme — sometimes explicit as in the empowerment chapters, and sometimes implicit, as in the public health chapter — underlying all social work practice is that of social control. The question of power and control, even in a system dedicated to making people well and preventing suffering, is critical. Issues of power begin with who controls expenditures and allocation for resources available for health care and end with the individual worker's power over those being served in their homes, in their communities, in hospitals and hospices.

Examples of the coercive power of health care systems are the mistreatment of psychiatric patients, enforced sterilisation or mutilation of selected populations, and treatments given without informed consent. Other examples are public health measures which may enforce isolation of those with certain diseases, such as those with tuberculosis in the early part of this century or those with HIV who are involuntarily detained in treatment programmes in contemporary Cuba.

Examples of 'positive power', assisting people to find and utilise their 'collective voice', were demonstrated in chapters 10 and 11 concerning work with those who have handicapping conditions. Implicitly, the public health framework focus on underserved and at-risk populations, often relies on community organisation and promotion of self-advocacy and self-help groups as empowering strategies which result in better access and better services to marginalised groups.

The power of medical personnel as a whole and medical staff as individuals was explored in the chapter on hospital social work (chapter 3).

Social Work Services in Health Settings:
Data from United States Manpower Studies

'Health social work' is the term used to refer to all of social work in the health field. It refers to the totality of the profession's contribution to both health and illness care. It is necessary, therefore, to address the question of what skills social workers must have in order to make contributions in health care and also to ask what content in professional education equips social workers (1) to work effectively in the health care sphere and (2) to deal with the problems and issues presented by patients, families and populations of those facing existing or potential health problems.

Patterns and content of studies leading to formal qualifications vary from country to country. In part, this reflects different systems of higher and vocational education. In part it reflects the different functions ascribed to social workers and different boundaries between social work and other professions and occupations. For example, in Germany the sozialarbeiter and sozialpadagoge exercise broadly similar functions (Barr, 1992). In Russia there is debate about the relationship of the emerging social work profession to that of social pedagogy (Bocharova, 1994). It is prudent to recognise this fact as the following discussion is based on the American experience.

In the United States, qualification for professional practice requires an undergraduate or postgraduate university degree in social work. In addition, there are those trained to provide social services in a wide variety of settings where demands of the job do not require the knowledge and skills acquired in professional education. Those preparing for these occupations are usually educated and trained in vocational schools and are typically referred to as 'social work assistants' or 'human service workers'.

Two large scale manpower studies have been done in the United States to determine what contributions university graduates with social work degrees make to the profession after entering the work-force. These data are necessary if the curriculum is to be relevant to the expectations in the work-place following professional education.

One study (Gibelman & Schervish, 1993) found that:

- 50 per cent of those with an undergraduate degree and 24 per cent of those with postgraduate degrees worked in primary settings serving those with severe health problems.
- 57 per cent listed mental health, medical clinics, ageing, substance abuse, developmental disabilities (for example, mental retardation, autism, cerebral palsy) and physical disabilities as their primary practice area.
- Hospitals and clinics ranked second as the primary setting for social work practice.
- 68 per cent of the sample were employed to provide direct service to clients as their primary function and nearly 43 per cent listed generalist social work as their practice speciality.

Another study (Teare & Sheafor) found:

- 45 per cent of undergraduates and 63 per cent of postgraduates listed hospitals, nursing homes/hospices, outpatient clinics, group/resident care homes, and psychiatric institutions as their employment settings — all settings dealing primarily with people who have serious health problems, chronic illness or handicapping conditions.
- Those with undergraduate degrees most often addressed health problems in generic social service agencies (such as municipal government offices, nursing homes, group homes and institutions).
- Postgraduates dominated jobs in specialised settings (such as mental health clinics, hospitals, schools, colleges, universities and private practice).
- Undergraduates needed skills required to assist their clients to deal with health-related problems but also skills related to helping clients obtain basic social provisions such as financial aid and housing.
- The data indicate that undergraduates appear to be more involved in 'caring for' clients and postgraduates in 'curing' individuals. Those with undergraduate degrees seem to help change situations that affect clients' social functioning. Those at postqualifying level are more clinical in their approach, rely more heavily on therapeutic models and techniques and tend to focus more on changing the person.

These studies clearly illustrate that a great proportion of social workers, in whatever setting they are employed, spend much of their time meeting the needs and solving the problems associated with clients who have, or are at risk of having, health problems. The data also indicate that (1) this is true regardless of level of training and (2) that these needs are addressed in a variety of general social service and specialist settings.

Curriculum Implications and Content

In modern times, the professional social worker would require skills needed (1) to help clients prevent the onset of illness and disability and (2) to help maintain optimum health of individuals, families, people at risk and (3) to enhance the ability of communities to provide a supportive social and ecologically sound environment.

The premise underlying all aspects of health social work is that the persons, families and organisations being served by the social worker are socially connected and that the central focus of the social worker in health care is these connections (Falck, 1988). The concept of 'connectedness' is inherent in the systems approach to social work practice and the generalist perspective outlined in chapter 1. The concept of connectedness also supports the view that because they are all part of a cultural system, health, illness and health care need to be understood in relation to each other. Health beliefs and behaviour, illness beliefs and behaviour and health care systems and activities are all governed by the same set of socially sanctioned rules in the context of a particular society (Currer & Stacy, 1986) so cultural understanding is an important aspect of any health-related curriculum.

Social work has historically been an 'integrating' profession so theories, concepts and research from a wide array of academic disciplines help inform and guide social work practice. These contributions need to be acknowledged and understood. Because of the profession's heavy reliance on social science content, some academicians view social work as 'applied social science'. Others view the essence of social work practice as being a mix of applied social science and the 'art' of helping people, this 'art' being dependent on humanistic values and understanding of the human condition gleaned from study of the humanities.

As far back as antiquity, health problems have been linked to economic, social and political conditions as well as to cultural factors. Six academic disciplines make significant contributions to understanding health and illness in modern times (Adler & Stone, 1979). These are summarised in Appendix A.

The manpower studies cited earlier in this chapter indicate that qualified social workers are providing services in a broad range of both generic and specialised social service agencies and serve people with a wide range of health problems and handicapping conditions.

Services provided in general social service agencies included obtaining concrete services (transportation, financial assistance) as well as indirect services (such as counselling, social support and problem solving).

Content for those offering social work services in general social service agencies needs to include:

- knowledge about health and illness with specific reference to the disease entities most apt to be encountered in the community or population being served;
- environmental factors which may affect health and illness;
- risk factors inherent in certain populations;
- activities which promote positive health and mental health;
- knowledge about mental illness;
- concepts of role theory and implications resulting from illness and/or disability;
- basic concepts from psychoanalytic crisis intervention and short-term task-centred casework; learning theory principles;
- functional and environmental assessment concepts;
- strategies for locating and/or developing community services and resources to meet existing needs of those with health-related problems;
- influence of culture on health and illness behaviour and on the health the health care system;
- environmental and attitudinal aspects related to non-compliance with medical regimens and impediments to effective utilisation of health care resources;
- interviewing skills sensitive to the self-image and self-esteem of those who are ill or disabled;
- understanding power relationships between physician, staff, patient, family and social worker;
- assessment of family situations and dynamics, especially as they have been affected by illness or disability of a family member;

- knowledge related to understanding of social support and natural helping systems;
- process-oriented skills related to development of social work intervention and roles appropriate to serving those who are ill or have handicapping conditions;
- advocacy and empowerment concepts as applied to social work practice with those who are ill or disabled;
- data collection skills and data analysis skills sufficient to contribute to self-assessment of one's own practice and to on-going assessment of social work's contributions to those being served.

Berkman has identified basic knowledge and competencies needed for beginning social work practice in a setting devoted entirely to health care (Berkman, 1985). These are listed in Table 1.(see page 209)

Those social workers in hospitals, clinics and other specialised settings tend to be trained at the post-qualifying level, where they focused more directly on the client than on the situation, tended to use more-formalised clinical interventions and are more apt to have administration and/or supervision as part of their responsibilities. This has a direct impact on curriculum content, and Table 2 (see page 210), adapted from Berkman, notes content necessary for advanced practice in health care settings.

The models of intervention which social workers need to examine include psychodynamic and crisis intervention models; behavioural and cognitive models; social psychological and communication models; systems and ecological models; and humanist and existential models.

These social workers will also need group facilitation skills and group treatment skills and knowledge of group dynamics. Because they will work in settings dominated by medical professionals, knowledge of medical ethics and ethical decision making becomes important. Advanced practice also implies sufficient leadership skills to engage in programme development and planning. Often this is dependent on some level of research ability and data analysis skills.

Social workers often become 'specialists' as a result of performing certain roles (for example, therapist, supervisor, administrator) or as a result of serving special populations (for example, cancer patients, children with leukaemia) or as a result of working in specialised settings (nursing homes, hospice, hospital, institution). As we have pointed out, however, this specialist knowledge usually builds on the generalist foundation acquired in the course of undergraduate training and the experience garnered in the practice setting.

Table 1 Basic Knowledge and Competencies Needed for Beginning Social Work Practice in Health Care

KNOWLEDGE BASE NEEDS	COMPETENCIES
1. Organisation of the health care system	— Awareness of various constituencies in health care and conflicting goals/demands social worker may encounter
2. Intra- and inter- professional and team practice and consultation; knowledge of group dynamics	— Ability to interview under difficult and uncertain conditions — Ability to ask appropriate questions of proper sources — Ability to communicate with a variety of professionals — Ability to work within team structure, contributing to decision making
3. Epidemiology of disease, including social environment risk factors	— Empathy and good listening skills — Ability to assess, evaluate and treat the illness situation as it relates to the family — Ability to understand experiences as reflected by different ages and types of patients
4. Social welfare entitlements and impact of legislation on practice (policy, administrative and regulatory)	— Awareness of health policy impact on social work services — Ability to interpret policy to patients family, other staff
5. Knowledge of impact of illness and psychosocial, economic and physical functioning of patient and family; including impact of diagnostic and treatment processes on the patient and family's life cycle; and awareness of stress producing elements in the course of treatment and rehabilitation	— Ability to complete a physical and psychosocial assessment covering the social and economic situation and other environment determinants — Ability to respond sensitively to cultural differences
6. Knowledge of transference and countertransference phenomena and their impact on the social worker as rationale for supervision and consultation	— Self awareness — Ability to manage anxiety — Ability to seek and utilise supervision and consultation

Adapted from Berkman and Carlton, 1985; used by permission

Table 2 Content for Advance Practice in Health Care

Organisation Dynamics in Health Care Settings and Institutional Change Strategies

Health, Disease and Illness with a Focus on Cultural Variations including natural and folk medicines's role in health beliefs

Social Health Policy: health care financing and delivery systems, mental health and long-term care of the elderly, chronically ill and disabled; concepts utilised in policy analysis

Specialised Practice Content Courses: Focus on Roles (advocacy, discharge planning, care management); ***Focus on Therapeutic Models*** (treatment-oriented group work, cognitive behavioural treatment, family systems and natural helping systems models, crisis intervention models, grief counselling and bereavement models, models of empowerment). ***Focus on Social Support and Self-help***

Stress, Crisis and transitions, with a focus on adaptive and maladaptive behaviour, the nature of stress, and factors in individual, family, and/or community that lead to or cause stress and affest adaptation and coping

Ethical Issues in Health Care: Focus on basic ethical theory combined with a problem solving approach to ethical issues confronted in the health arena and integrated into the social work practice ehtical standards

In-depth Process Knowledge and skills needed for leadership, programme development, planning, consultation, supervision and teaching

Management Concepts and application in health care

Research Design and Utilisation and application to health concerns and systems; abilities in epidemiological and prevention-oriented research

Adapted from Berkman and Carlton, 1985; used by permission

At both undergraduate and postgraduate levels of training the concepts of role, stress and adaptation, coping and social support should be a central emphasis in the curriculum.

Conclusion, Reflections and Challenges

All industrialised countries are faced with limited resources to meet the health care needs of a rapidly expanding and ageing population — a population which, because of technological advances, longer life-spans, and contamination from environmental hazards, increasingly lives with long-term illness and severely handicapping conditions. Governments and the public therefore ask, 'Are we getting benefits for the expenditures being made in health care?' In other words, what is the outcome accruing from the investment made in health care generally and, for the purpose of this chapter, in social workers' involvement in health care?

These questions demand that data be furnished which show that social work makes a difference in a health care environment that (1) is increasingly oriented to the positive of social health rather than a disease-focused model of health, (2) uses people's strengths instead of focusing on their weaknesses, (3) educates the populace for health maintenance and health promotion and (4) helps prevent illness. Under these conditions, the profession of social work will have to become adept at outcome research and cost:benefit analysis. The profession will also have to identify strategies which develop programmes not reliant on government funding. Developing and working with non-governmental organisations is one such strategy. Mobilising volunteer resources and supporting self-advocacy and self-help groups are two other such strategies.

Two issues deserve special mention: (1) the health care system in the United States has the faith of the people who can afford insurance; the problem is not quality of care but the high cost of high technology care and the inaccessibility of care to uninsured people; (2) the health care system is undergoing rapid change rather than diminishing in size and scope.

In relation to these same two issues in the former Soviet Union and eastern Europe one can say that (1) because of recent shortages in supplies and technology, many have lost faith in the health care system and (2) the health care systems that were part of the Soviet Union are also rapidly changing. However in view of past underfunding of the state system of medical care, there is tremendous pressure to expand the system and level of care with little by way of increased resources.

Both sets of circumstances have implications for social work. Social workers in the United States must increasingly operate within cost controls, eligibility requirements and increasingly complex bureaucratic structures. They must assume a strong advocacy stance on behalf of their clients who have health-related problems. They must also adjust to a health care system that is increasingly fragmented and relate to new types of programmes which may be untested for reliability and quality.

Social workers in eastern Europe and former Soviet states may face greater demands for educating patients about the health care system and helping patients develop ways of assessing the adequacy of the services they are receiving and speaking out for services that are needed. Prevention-oriented education done at the community level may also be recognised as of a higher importance — education aimed at keeping people healthier so they make fewer demands on an already underfunded medical service.

They may also face the necessity of helping medical services extend their programmes without increasing their costs. As an example, social workers might spend time organising volunteers who would provide services that would make health-care settings more humane (for example, setting up volunteers to visit patients who are far from home or have no families or assisting families of hospital patients with temporary housing arrangements). Such volunteer activities enhance the community's knowledge of and commitment to health-related agencies and at the same time extend their services and make the environment more humane and comfortable.

Social workers might also help establish non-profit charitable organisations within hospitals, hospices, nursing homes and clinics. Their function would be to organise fund-raising events and, by so doing, increase community education and awareness. Such activities would be considered community development and fulfil the social worker's role as community organiser and resource developer.

Professionally trained social workers in many countries face challenges in the following areas: (1) effective arrangements for long-term care of those with chronic illness and frail elderly people; (2) community-based care for those with severe mental illness and severe learning difficulties; (3) situations concerning cost and effectiveness of social work services; (4) producing useful and methodologically sound research which contributes to better outcomes; (5) ability to contribute to the design of social planning and social policy.

It is evident that social work practice in the health care sphere operates in the midst of considerable tensions between major political, economic and social systems. The issues are change v. stability, individual v. collective rights, radical reform v. rejuvenation of health care systems, facilitation v. restriction of access to health care.

Social change does not occur when systems are in a state of stability but when broad changes in social conditions bring about recognition of the need for changes in response to society's problems. Changes occur in times of ideological conflicts, the changing plight of oppressed populations, and major disruption of personal relationships in families, groups and communities (Netting *et al.*, 1993).

In today's environment, which is characterised by such rapid social change, professionally trained social work practitioners are compelled to recognise the influence of politics and power on their practice and seize the opportunities posed by changing conditions and challenges to improve the situations of life of those they serve. For those social work practitioners whose practice focuses on health-related issues, this means finding ways to improve the situations of life of those driven to the margins of society because of poor health or handicapping conditions.

Political understanding is essential in a social work practice which addresses numerous constraints and opportunities. Sometimes a single incident (such as the Chernobyl disaster or the Kobe earthquake or the Los Angeles race riots) or a developing social movement (such as the environmental movement or the consumer:users' movement) can cause monolithic systems to fluctuate. Political and power systems in much of the world today are characterised by such fluctuations. These fluctuations do not necessarily lead to revolutions, but discussions and actions taken in the midst of such fluctuations may result in new ideas, new movements and new conditions being accepted by the established political and power structures (Ryan & Gordon, 1994).

'The problem of the "body" . . . raises in acute form the whole debate on the relationship between mind and body, culture and nature, self and society' (Turner, 1987). The effective professionally trained social worker therefore needs a complex cognitive map to help grasp a complex world, the complex situations of those being helped and the complex systems which attempt to offer hope and help. This cognitive map must be based on a view of professional practice that recognises both the *possibilities* and *constraints* on practice. Such a map must recognise the *interplay between politics and power* and the *interdependency of social policy and social work practice* (Rees, 1991). It requires a macrosociological view of social structures, political processes and economic conditions — all of which in various complex ways shape the nature of health in modern societies (Turner, 1987).

Following Talcott Parsons's and Richard Titmuss's work on the sociology of the professions in the 1950s and 1960s, there was considerable unease over the use of 'power' by professional èlites. Contemporary sociologists are more likely to view professionalisation as a growth in power and status (Turner, 1987) resting on a defined body of knowledge, accountability to the public, a subscribed set of values, a code of ethical behaviour, and a structure of professional accreditation and imposed sanctions.

Power is always an issue in professional practice. In part, the power of a profession rests on its members' ability to make claims successfully about the scientific value of their work and the way in which their professional knowledge is grounded in precise, accurate and reliable scientific information. For social work, this type of power accrues from the applied social science aspects of its profession.

In part, the power of a profession rests on its ability to change for the better the lives of those it serves. For social work, this power accrues directly from the success of advocacy, ability to influence social policy, and giving voice to the collectives being served.

Social work practitioners dealing with today's health care systems face situations where there are power conflicts between lay groups and professional groups, between governments and non-governmental organisations, between competing economic structures and theories. Practitioners therefore need a perspective on health care which can effect reconciliation or successful resolution of these conflicts.

Rees addresses this issue when he suggests that the means of simultaneously addressing individual problems and social issues lies in 'the promise of biography'. The proposition is that as a result of telling their story, people see themselves in a different light and from having others listen to their accounts, they build a political analysis and identity. Politics becomes, in this sense, an understanding that politics and power are concerned with day-to-day relationships as well as competition over scarce resources in an organisation or a society.

Social workers must engage in this 'power process' in two ways: (1) they facilitate '*giving voice*' to individuals and groups, by harnessing their energy for the realisation of their common aspirations and (2) they also engage in this 'power process' by '*being a voice*', a collective professional voice, for those unable or unwilling to speak for themselves.

In this sense, power has little to do with authoritarianism and much to do with facilitating, enabling, educating and democratising. It has to do with social justice and tackling the issues of social injustice. Achieving power in Rees's model demands humility, political skills, assertiveness, and willingness to listen to those who have been ignored, undervalued, marginalised. In terms of health care, this means those elements of populations who have long term illnesses, have handicapping conditions, and those denied a basic level of health care.

Preparing Social Workers for Practice in Health Care

Social work is an international profession. Throughout the world social work colleagues work with others to face enormous health problems in the 'global community': (1) serving an increasingly frail, elderly population; (2) dealing with great changes in family structure that have enormous implications for dependent people; (3) combating new diseases, such as AIDS; (4) coping with the impact of environmental degradation on health status; (5) facing increasing levels of violence in societies; (6) coping with the toll on health taken by urbanisation; (7) attempting to change economic policies which are plunging increasing numbers of people into poverty and depriving them of basic nutrition and health care.

As members of an international profession we have both a great opportunity and a great responsibility to learn from each other. In terms of health care, we need to share accounts of how individuals are conscious of their sickness or wellness, how knowledge of health and illness are constituted in the everyday lives of those we serve and the everyday life of professional practice in the health care sphere. We must ascertain how, and if, those with health problems are treated in a humane way. We must try to abstract from our work in health care a kind of comprehensive narrative of what's happening in health care both locally and globally. This means a commitment to sharing each other's successes as well as failures, communicating our experiences through research and publications and conferences. It means finding new ways to communicate with each other via information technology (such as internet and electronic mail). We need the will and the commitment to do this as we move toward the challenges facing health care systems in the twenty-first century.

Systems under stress may become heavily bureaucratic and authoritarian and may dehumanise the very individuals and groups they aim to serve. In the twenty-first century, social workers everywhere face the challenges of fostering humane practices which recognise the strengths of those who are ill or marginalised; promoting environments which foster health; and building programmes which humanise both those providing services and those who receive them.

References

Adler, Nancy and Stone, George; 'Social Science Perspectives on the Health System' in *Health Psychology* (eds) Stone, G., Cohen, F. and Adler, Nancy; (1979) London; Jossey-Bass.

Barr, Hugh; *In Europe: Social Work Education and 1992*; (1992) London, Central Council for Education and Training in Social Work.

Berkman, Barbara; in *The Development of Health Social Work Curricula;* (eds) Berkman, Barbara and Carlton, T O (1985) Boston, MGH Institute of Health Professionals.

Bocharova, Valentina; NASW; in press.

Carlton, T O; *Clinical Health Settings*; (1984) NY, Springer.

Currer, Caroline and Stacy, Margaret (eds) (1986) *Concepts of Health, Illness and Disease*; NY; Berg.

Falck, Hans S (1988)*Social Work: The Membership Perspective*; Springer.

Rees, Stuart; *Achieving Power; Practice and Policy in Social Welfare* (1991) Allen & Unwin, Australia.

Ryan, M. and Gordon, A. (eds); *Body Politics: Disease, Desire and the Family*, (1994) Westview Press, Oxford.

Teare, Robt. J. and Sheafor, Bradford W., 'National Task Analysis of Analysis Study of Social Work Practice'; unpublished manuscript, Tuscaloosa: University of Alabama School of Social Work; used by permission of the authors.

Turner, Bryan S.; *Medical Power and Social Knowledge*; (1987) Sage Publications, London.

Appendix A
Disciplinary Contributions to Perspectives on Health Care

DISCIPLINE	CONTRIBUTIONS	RESEARCH METHODS
Applied Anthropology	— Disruption of traditional cultures as stress factor in development of health problems — Adaptiveness of human systems' responses to environmental stress — Curative activities of traditional healers — Meanings of health care activities to providers and receivers of service — Cross-cultural training of health workers	— Epidemiology — Ethnographic — Qualitative
Economics	— Macro-level interactions between health seekers and health care providers — How control is exercised by professionals — Access to health care — Effectiveness of providers in terms of morbidity and mortality — Organisational power struggles for control over resource — Decision making in health care settings concerning resource allocation	— Large scale systems and data analysis — Statistical analysis — Mathematical modelling — Organisation Development Analysis
Medical Sociology (formerly social medicine)	— Medicine as a social institution — Illness as deviance — Medicine as profession — Social class differences in health status — Social aetiology and ecology of disease — Study of medical treatment and recovery — Impact of new technology — Examines assumptions of economic models of health	— Behaviour of participants in health care sphere as influenced by adaptive needs, social demands, situational pressures — Large scale systems analysis — Surveys — Statistical analysis
Medicine ● Psychiatry	— Clinical case management — Psychotherapy effectiveness — Basic research on biological processes	— Case studies — Statistical analysis — Laboratory